Springer Japan KK

N. Chino · J.L. Melvin (Eds.)

Functional Evaluation of Stroke Patients

With 54 Figures

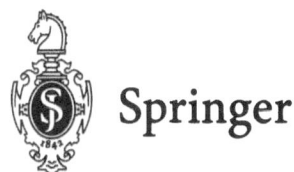

Springer

Editors

Naoichi Chino, M.D., M.S., D.M.Sc.
Professor and Chairman
Department of Rehabilitation Medicine
Keio University School of Medicine
Tokyo, Japan

John L. Melvin, M.D., M.M.Sc.
Professor and Deputy Chairman
Department of Physical Medicine and
Rehabilitation, Temple University,
Pennsylvania, USA

Associate Editors

Murray E. Brandstater, M.B.B.S., Ph. D.,
F.R.C.P.(C)
Professor and Chairman
Department of Physical Medicine and
Rehabilitation
Loma Linda University,
California, USA

Carl V. Granger, M.D.
Professor and Director
Center for Functional Assessment Research
Department of Rehabilitation Medicine
School of Medicine and Biomedical Sciences
State University of New York at Buffalo
New York, USA

Prof. Dr. med Karl-Heinz Mauritz
Klinik Berlin, Department of Neurological
Rehabilitation, Free University Berlin,
Berlin, Germany

ISBN 978-4-431-68463-3
DOI 10.1007/978-4-431-68461-9

ISBN 978-4-431-68461-9 (eBook)

Printed on acid-free paper

© Springer Japan 1996
Originally published by Springer-Verlag Tokyo 1996
Softcover reprint of the hardcover 1st edition 1996

Typesetting: Best-set Typesetter Ltd., Hong Kong

Preface

Stroke is one of the major causes of disability in the world. Consequently, an effective rehabilitation regimen is the goal of specialists working in the field worldwide. The implementation of rehabilitation programs for the stroke patient is broad in scope and requires, first of all, an objective scientific evaluation method.

In 1980 the World Health Organization developed the International Classification of Impairments, Disabilities, and Handicaps. It categorized impairments and disabilities on the basis of functional evaluation but took into account cultural and socioeconomic factors when defining handicaps, thus making it difficult to use the same functional evaluation instrument for the three phenomena.

In this monograph, experts in the treatment of stroke from Japan, the United States, and Europe share their ideas presented during the 31st Annual Convention of the Japanese Association of Rehabilitation Medicine held in June 1994. All the participants freely contributed their views on the functional assessment and prognosis of stroke patients. Indeed, their contributions shed light on possible breakthroughs in the future for the development of rehabilitation regimens for stroke patients.

November 1995   Naoichi Chino
                                                         John L. Melvin

Acknowledgments

The authors of this monograph express their thanks to the following organizing committee members:

Kazuo Akaboshi, Motohide Arita, Hiroki Ebata, Toshiyuki Fujiwara, Kozo Hanayama, Yukihiro Hara, Kimitaka Hase, Fujiko Hotta, Shin-ichi Izumi, Suminori Kawakami, Ken Kondoh, Kunitsugu Kondoh, Yoshihisa Masakado, Kiyoshi Mineo, Tomoko Misawa, Eiji Mori, Masaaki Nagata, Yukio Noda, Yoshihisa Nunotani, Tetsuo Ohta, Yasutomo Okajima, Tomokichi Otsuka, Masaru Seki, Hidetoshi Takahashi, Morimasa Takahashi, Masako Takayama, Naofumi Tanaka, Hiroyuki Toikawa, Tetsuya Tomaru, Akio Tsubahara, Tetsuya Tsuji, and Kazuo Tsujiuchi.

This symposium was sponsored in part by the Pfizer Health Research Foundation.

Contents

List of Contributors

Adachi, T.   115

Brandstater, M. E.   9, 93

Chino, N.   19, 33, 103

Denzler, P. E.   45
Domen, K.   19, 33, 103

Fiedler, R. C.   75
Findley, T. W.   59

Granger, C. V.   75

Hesse, S.   45

Ishigami, S.   125

Johnston, M. V.   59

Kimura, A.   19, 33

Liu, M.   125

Maney, M.   59
Mauritz, K.-H.   45
Melvin, J. L.   1

Saitoh, E.   19, 33, 103
Sonoda, S.   19, 33, 103

Whyte, J.   1

Zorowitz, R. D.   59

Evaluation of Stroke: A Review

John L. Melvin[1,2] *and John Whyte*[1,2]

Summary. A comprehensive review of evaluation issues related to stroke would require more than a short chapter. However, the subject is of great importance. Stroke
is the most frequent cause of death in the United States. Health care and lost productivity costs associated with stroke reached an estimated 15.6 billion dollars in the
United States in 1991. Despite these significant impacts, clinicians in the United States
often treat similar stroke patients quite differently. This suggests that greater uniformity in evaluation and treatment could result in better clinical outcomes and economic efficiency. To accomplish these goals, evaluation of stroke patients requires the
development of a patient database that includes information categorized as in the
International Classification of Impairment, Disability, and Handicap. Additionally it
should include medical and quality-of-life information. Information regarding these
conceptually different categories permits the development of appropriate strategies
for their treatment and the framework to evaluate their outcomes. These categories
also permit facilities to compare their results against others. Although clinicians focus
primarily on medical and functional outcomes, organizations responsible for health
care increasingly include patient and family satisfaction and cost efficiency as measures of effectiveness. Those performing evaluations select their measurement instruments on the basis of sensibility, validity, reliability, and sensitivity. A number of
examinations, instruments, and scales provide appropriate information regarding the
pathology, impairment, disability, handicap, and quality of life of stroke patients. This
will increasingly become the foundation of clinical practice as outcome analysis influences which treatments may be utilized in the treatment of stroke.

Introduction

A full discussion of the evaluation issues related to stroke would be a task beyond the
scope of a short chapter. The presentation of stroke varies widely, not only in its
pathology but also in the resulting permanent neurological impairment, disability,

---

[1]MossRehab Hospital and The Moss Rehabilitation Research Institute, 1200 West Tabor Road,
Philadelphia, PA 19141-3099, USA
[2]Temple University, Department of Physical Medicine and Rehabilitation, 3401 N. Broad St.,
Philadelphia, PA 19140, USA

and handicap [1]. The relationships among these hierarchical concepts are themselves complex, further adding to the difficulty of presenting a full discussion of evaluation. Thus, this chapter is limited to alerting clinicians to the need to improve evaluation procedures, outlining the goals to be achieved by evaluation, presenting promising measurement tools, and recommending approaches to evaluation likely to keep the assessments of clinicians effective, efficient, and contemporary.

Need to Review Stroke Evaluation

Clinicians in rehabilitation medicine begin evaluating stroke patients early in their training. Most continue to do so regularly thereafter. Thus, some might question the need to discuss evaluation in a monograph targeted for rehabilitation clinicians. However, the magnitude of the impact of stroke on patients and society combined with increased economic restrictions on health care makes such a review timely and imperative. Stroke is a problem of such size that relatively small increases in treatment effectiveness and efficiency could significantly improve patient lives and save millions of dollars in social costs.

In the United States, stroke is the third most frequent cause of death; approximately 500 000 strokes per year result in 150 000 deaths [2]. The American Heart Association [2] estimates that the United States has 3 million stroke survivors, many of whom have significant impairment and disability. The consequences of these strokes on individuals and their families can be significant as they may go beyond physical dependence to changes in role relationships, social isolation, and financial crisis. The impacts of stroke go beyond the personal consequences on patients and their families. From a social point of view, the economic impact is tremendous. Health care and lost productivity costs reached an estimated 15.6 billion dollars in the United States in 1991 [2]. Health care costs alone are significant. Stroke is the largest category of patients admitted to rehabilitation hospitals [3]. The increase in number of rehabilitation hospitals has been substantial, from 357 in 1984 to 812 in 1990. These facilities cost 14 billion dollars per year [4].

Stroke patients with no apparent differences are treated in a highly variable fashion. Survivors are discharged to a number of post acute care options including home health care, skilled nursing facilities, rehabilitation hospitals, and nursing homes with limited evidence of facility-specific influences on outcomes [5]. Admission rates to rehabilitation hospitals vary widely. In a three-city study, for instance, admission rates varied from 11% to 20% [5]. This same study showed that use of home health care varied from 20% to 38% and that of skilled nursing facilities from 10% to 36% [5]. This suggests the need to identify inequitable or inefficient approaches.

Another reason to reexamine the information available from stroke evaluation is the need to strengthen the case for stroke rehabilitation. Most papers addressing this question are descriptive in nature rather than conforming to a disciplined experimental design. As a result, there are legitimate questions as to how much improvement occurs through spontaneous recovery, how much functional adaptation might occur through informal mechanisms, and how much can be attributed to specific rehabilitation treatment.

This questioning occurs at a time when the scarcity of resources available for human services includes health care. Thus, any service without a strong research-supported rationale is vulnerable to restrictions.

Goals of Stroke Evaluation

The primary goal of evaluation is to describe patients and their circumstances through the development of a patient database. Such a database has value to the extent that it can be used in making decisions regarding patient care, suggesting that information must be useful in decision making if it is to be collected. It also suggests the need for sufficient information to make the decisions necessary for the care of stroke patients. Medical evaluations traditionally have limited the quantity of the information they obtained regarding function and quality of life, and even many rehabilitation practitioners have been less than thorough or have lacked systematic approaches to these questions. To develop effective rehabilitation treatment plans, however, the database must describe all aspects of patients.

It is therefore important that the patient database address questions of pathology, impairment (absence or altered function of an organ or system), disability (altered ability to perform an activity in a manner considered normal), and handicap (the disadvantage that an individual experiences as a result of an impairment or disability limiting or preventing the exercise of a normal social role) [1]. Information regarding each of these conceptually different categories permits the development of appropriate strategies for their treatment. The database should also include information regarding associated medical complications and comorbidities as these may have prognostic significance [6].

Finally, quality-of-life information should be collected. While needing further refinement, the concept of quality of life includes such factors as ability to perform social roles; physical, emotional, economic, and subjective health status; capacity for social interaction; and intellectual functioning. Its improvement is becoming an accepted goal of health care professionals [7], reflecting their awareness that these outcomes are those that matter most to patients and their families.

A complete database provides the information needed to determine appropriate care. Necessary decisions include whether rehabilitation services of any type are needed, which setting is most appropriate for the needed services, and what specific services are needed. Additional decisions include to what extent treatment decisions target the needs of patients through focusing on the patients themselves, their caregivers, or their physical and social environments.

Many stroke programs currently organize their evaluations to provide explicit information at intervals regarding the status of patients, the treatment they have received, and the level of preparedness of their caregivers for their discharge. These interval measurements of patient status allow documentation of individual patient progress. They also provide the data that can be used to compare effectiveness among institutions. Facilities can thus compare their success to others treating similar patients. The Uniform Data System (UDS) of the State University of New York (Buffalo), utilizing the Functional Independence Measures (FIM) is the program most commonly used in the United State for such interfacility comparisons [8]. Such approaches depend on the ability to identify comparable classes of patients. Many rehabilitation professionals believe that case-mix measures need further development to allow comparisons to be made with greater validity, reliability, and sensitivity.

Increasingly, evaluations are used to identify the outcomes resulting after rehabilitation treatment. These include measures of patient status, satisfaction of patients and their families, and costs or resources used, particularly as compared to functional gains. These outcomes increasingly are time related to the onset of the stroke rather than occurring only at the time of discharge from the rehabilitation hospital or unit.

An emerging use of evaluations is to classify patients into prospectively developed categories. This technique looks for characteristics that permit groupings of patients in a search for standardization rather than looking at the unique differences among patients. These patient categories can be used to determine the type of facility from which patients will receive rehabilitation care, permit predictions of resource needs, suggest appropriate clinical pathways, and identify expected outcomes. Most of these classification tools remain to be developed. However, a system is currently being developed by Margaret Stineman of the University of Pennsylvania that permits rehabilitation hospital length of stay to be predicted from patient classification. The elements of this classification include FIM impairment category, admission FIM score, and age. This approach has become known as the Function Related Groups (FRGs) system. The FRGs have been developed after extensive research. In contrast, some rehabilitation systems move patients to facilities of differing intensity of care through the use of pragmatically derived patient classification systems. These are usually also based on FIM scores. It is reasonable to assume more such classification techniques will be used as managed care becomes more extensively used in the United States.

Characteristics of Evaluation Measures

The success of evaluation measures used in clinical evaluation relates to their sensibility, reliability, validity, and sensitivity. For clinical measures to be used successfully, they must substantively reflect these characteristics.

Sensibility refers to the reasonableness of using a measure. This in turn is determined by there being an important purpose for its inclusion and relative ease of its use.

Validity is an index as to how well any evaluation tool actually measures what it purports to measure. In the context of this discussion, predictive validity becomes important; that is, how well does the performance of an evaluation measure predict future performance of a real-life task?

Reliability refers to the ability of two different individuals to achieve similar results or the ability of a single individual to obtain similar results when administering the evaluation instrument on two separate occasions.

Sensitivity refers to the capacity of a clinical evaluation tool to reflect important changes. Each of these measures requires a value judgment as to whether the results of the underlying measure are useful.

Measurement Instruments

This section identifies specific measurement instruments capable of providing valid and reliable assessments of pathology, impairment, disability, handicap, and related concepts. Because stroke patients may demonstrate cognitive or linguistic impairment, use of these assessment instruments may require confirmation of their comprehension and the reliability of their responses. This may be done by repeating a subset of questions in the evaluation instrument to confirm that the patient provides consistent responses. In addition, caregiver proxy data may be given for questions the patient cannot answer directly. The validity of caregiver proxy data varies from measure to measure, and its use requires further study. Despite these accommodations, there may be some subjects who cannot answer and will have missing data from some of the measures.

Pathology

The medical and neurological examinations are the best means of identifying comorbid diseases and the clinical manifestations of stroke. The pattern of these manifestations may be useful in localizing the pathological lesion. However, neuroimaging studies provide a more specific way of identifying neural structures involved as well as the most probable vascular territory of an infarct. Other studies during the acute phase may be useful to establish the etiology of stroke or to assess changes of the patient's condition or complications.

Impairment

Motor impairments such as dysarthria, impaired movement of the arms, legs, and face, and ataxia can all be assessed by the National Institute of Health (NIH) stroke scale. [9] This scale documents neurological impairment in acute stroke. Its interrater and test–retest reliability are high. The scale has undergone extensive testing for validity.

Detailed evaluation of motor function can be assessed with the impairment scale of the Chedoke-McMaster Stroke Assessment (C-MSA). It includes items on shoulder pain, postural control, and movement of the arm, leg, and foot [10,11]. Proprioception in the upper extremities may be assessed with the Thumb Finding Test [12]. Cognitive function can be evaluated using the Neurobehavioral Cognitive Status Examination (NCSE), which is a standardized assessment of cognitive function. It is scored in several domains. Its appropriateness and ease of use for stroke patients has been well documented [13,14].

Disability

Many facilities in the United States utilize the FIM as a basic measure of disability [9]. This instrument includes scales measuring self-care, sphincter control, mobility, loco-motion, communication, and social cognition.

In the context of thorough evaluation, the authors believe the FIM should be supplemented in the areas of cognition and communication. An indication of gait efficiency can be determined by measuring the amount of time required for the patient to walk 10 m in those capable of doing so [15].

Functional communication skills can be assessed by the Communicative Effectiveness Index (CETI), which requires responses to 16 items about the patient's performance in everyday situations [16]. It has demonstrated an acceptable level of validity and reliability [17].

Advanced (instrumental) activities of daily living can be measured by the Frenchay Activities Index (FAI), which has been validated for stroke patients and is a measure often used for everyday activities [18].

Handicap

The elements needed to assess handicap include both the types of roles the patient assumes and the environmental factors that support or impede fulfillment of these roles. The Craig Handicap Assessment and Reporting Technique (CHART) is emerging as a significant tool for the measurement of handicap. It focuses on the frequency of activities that are defined by a spectrum of social roles, including work [19]. Its author is currently conducting trials with stroke patients to determine if the same reliability and validity noted in spinal cord injury patients can be applied to the stroke population.

Quality of Life

As discussed earlier, quality of life is a multifaceted construct that cannot be measured by a single scale. It is a product of many factors in addition to health and functional capacity.

Poor emotional coping may have a profound impact on activity levels, resulting in a diminished quality of life. The Center for Epidemiologic Studies–Depression scale (CES-D) has been validated in clinical and nonclinical samples [20,21]. It compares favorably with other depression scales and has been successfully applied to stroke populations. [22].

Another measure of quality of life is the Short Form-36 (SF-36). It has been widely used to survey health status after its development by the investigators of the Medical Outcomes Study [23]. It appears to be appropriate for stroke patients [24].

Life satisfaction can be measured by the seven-point Faces Scale. This is a nonverbal scale shown to have excellent validity in a wide range of settings [25,26]. In older stroke patients, the Life Satisfaction Index-A (LSI-A) can be used to explore the general feelings of well-being among older people [27]. It has been more thoroughly evaluated than other life satisfaction scales [26].

Caregiver Evaluation

The same scales utilized to measure quality of life in those with stroke can be given to their caregivers to answer from their own perspectives. Caregivers also can be given the FAI, the CHART, and the Questionnaire on Resources and Stress [28], which explores attitudes toward the patient, time and financial burdens of patient care, and concerns about the patient's future.

This listing of measurement instruments focuses attention on the extensive information necessary to adequately follow the stroke patient and provide for treatment programs that result in optimal quality of life for stroke patients and their families. While the need for most of this information probably is known to rehabilitation treatment teams, it rarely is collected systematically or in a form that facilitates valid and reliable retrieval. The validity of many of these scales in those with cognitive deficits is unknown. Their usefulness in such circumstances should be explored. To achieve the goals of systematic collection and appropriate retrieval will require the careful design of information systems that facilitate systematic care. Much work remains to be done to make this practical within the clinical setting.

Clinical Recommendations

The authors have a number of recommendations for those who wish to prepare themselves for the practice models likely to emerge in the future.

1. Systematize the collection of data: all stroke clinicians currently collect information but few present it in a systematic, consistent, and retrievable fashion. Begin these habits to prepare for the information-based practice of the future.
2. Computerize where possible: facilitate the collection, display, and retrieval of information through standardized techniques with computer support.
3. Use standardized scales: to the extent possible, integrate a number of standardized scales into the information your clinical teams collect. Attempt to substitute the elements of the scales for information currently collected rather than adding information.
4. Compare if possible with others: begin to use national and international comparative databases that allow benchmarking, that is, comparing your performance against that of others.
5. Think prospectively: integrate prospectively developed protocols into your practice. Establish expected outcomes and treatment protocols (clinical pathways) to match specific categories of patients. Organize these in ways to be able to predict the expected cost to achieve significant clinical outcomes.
6. Monitor repetitively: within your information systems and treatment protocols, incorporate decision points where outcomes, treatment delivered, and costs are reviewed to identify progress and initiate corrective action where necessary.
7. Achieve community outcomes: focus rehabilitation efforts toward maximizing function and quality of life in the community setting through measuring rehabilitation outcomes at specific times after community reintegration.
8. Be cost-effective: recognize that the resources for health care and human services are limited. Develop methods of achieving comparable outcomes with as few resources as possible.
9. Reevaluate clinical protocols: be prepared at consistent intervals to review your treatment system so as to constantly improve it.
10. Adopt advances: develop a mechanism to keep abreast of new approaches that promise to be more effective and efficient. As they occur, incorporate them into your own systems.

By working incrementally toward these goals, clinicians can position themselves to improve their services and adapt to future changes in practice.

References

1. World Health Organization (WHO) (1980) International classification of impairments, disabilities, and handicaps (ICDIDH). WHO, Geneva, Switzerland
2. American Heart Association (1991) Heart and stroke facts. American Heart Association, Washington, DC
3. Hosek S, Kane R, Carney M, Hartman J, Reboussin D, Serato C, Melvin JL (1986) Charges and outcomes for rehabilitative care, implications for the prospective payment system. RAND/UCLA Center for Health Care Financing Policy Research (R-3424-HFCA), University of California, Los Angeles

4. ProPAC (1991) Report to Congress: U.S. Government Printing Office, Washington
5. University of Minnesota School of Public Health, Institute of Health (1993) A final report: post acute care (HFCA #17-C98891). University of Minnesota, Minneapolis, Table 24
6. Jameison DG (1991) Acute management of the stroke patient. Phys Med Rehabil Clin North Am 2:437
7. Levine S (1977) The changing terrains in medical sociology: emergent concern with quality of life. J Health Soc Behav 28:1–6
8. Hamilton BB, Granger CV, Sherwin FS, Zielezny M, Tashman JS (1986) A uniform national data system for medical rehabilitation. Rehabilitation Outcomes. Paul H, Brookes Publishing, Baltimore
9. Brott T, Marler JR, Olinger CP, et al (1989) Measurements of acute cerebral infarction: a clinical examination scale. Stroke 20:864–870
10. Twitchell TE (1951) The restoration of motor function following hemiplegia in man. Brain 74:443–480
11. Brunnstrom S (1970) Movement therapy in hemiplegia: a neuropsychological approach. Harper and Row, New York
12. Prescott RJ, Garraway WM, Ahktar AJ (1982) Predicting functional outcome following acute stroke using a standard clinical examination. Stroke 13:641–644
13. Kierman RJ, Mueller J, Langston JW, VanDyke C (1987) The neurobehavioral cognitive status examination: a brief but differentiated approach to cognitive assessment. Ann Intern Med 107:481–485
14. Osman DC, Smet IC, Winegarden B, Gandhavadi B (1992) Neurobehavioral cognitive status examination: its use with unilateral stroke patients in a rehabilitation setting. Arch Phys Med Rehabil 73:414–418
15. Wade DT, Wood VA, Heller A, et al (1987) Walking after stroke: measurement and recovery over the first three months. Scand J Rehabil Med 19:25–30
16. Lomas J, Laura P, Bester S, Elbard H, Finlayson A, Zogheib C (1989) The communicative effectivenes index: development and psychometric evaluation of a functional communication measure for adult aphasia. J Speech Hear Disord 54:113–124
17. Manochiopinig S, Sheard C, Reed VA (1992) Pragmatic assessment in adult aphasia: a clinical review. Aphasiology 6:519–533
18. Holbrook M, Skilbeck CE (1983) An activities index for use with stroke patients. Age Aging 12:166–170
19. Whiteneck GG, Charlifue MA, Gerhart KA, Overholser JD, Richardson GN (1992) Quantifying handicaps: a new measure of long-term rehabilitation outcomes. Arch Phys Med Rehabil 73:519–526
20. Randloff LS (1977) The CES-D Scale: a self-report depression scale for research in the general population. Appl Psychol Meas 1:385–401
21. Himmelfarb S, Murrell SA (1983) Reliability and validity of five mental health scales in older persons. J Gerentol 38:333–334
22. Robinson RG, Boldue PL, Price TR (1987) Two-year longitudinal study of post mood stroke disorders: diagnosis and outcome at one and two years. Stroke 18:837–843
23. Ware JE, Sherbourne CD (1992) The MOS 36 Item Short Form Health Survey. I. Conceptual framework and item selection. Med Care 30:473–481
24. DeHaan R, Aaronson N, Limburg M, Langton HR, van Crevel H (1993) Measuring quality of life in stroke. Stroke 24:320–327
25. Andrews FM, Crandall R (1976) The validity of measures of self-reported well being. Soc Indicat Res 3:1–19
26. McDowell I, Newell C (1987) Measuring health: a guide to rating scales and questionnaires. Oxford, New York
27. Neugarten BL, Havighurst RJ, Tobin SS (1961) The measurement of life satisfaction. J Gerontol 16:134–143
28. Holroyd J (1987) Questionnaire on resources and stress. Clinical Psychology Publishing, Brandon

Basic Aspects of Impairment Evaluation in Stroke Patients

Murray E. Brandstater[1]

Summary. Focal brain lesions caused by stroke confer on the patient a set of neurological deficits. These deficits are called impairments. Evaluation of these impairments constitutes an essential first step in management of the patient. In the acute patient, evaluation of the impairments helps the physician determine the pathology, localization, and severity of the lesion. For rehabilitation, evaluation of the impairments helps the clinician determine functional prognosis, establish rehabilitation goals, and define the treatment program. The key neurological impairments observed in stroke patients may be grouped under the following headings: mental status, communication, cranial nerves, motor function, sensory function, and posture and balance. Evaluation methods for some of the deficits have been refined through the development of scaled tests, allowing quantification. Use of scores from scaled tests allows the clinician to rate severity of the impairment and to monitor recovery.

Introduction

The focal neurological lesion that accompanies the clinical syndrome recognized as a stroke confers on the patient a set of neurological deficits. In rehabilitation medicine, these deficits are referred to as impairments. The initial responsibility of the physician is to establish the diagnosis, which involves defining the pathology and the neurological deficits (Table 1). The physician is then able to prescribe specific therapy. For rehabilitation of a stroke patient, the identification, characterization, and measurement of impairments are analogous to establishing a diagnosis. Evaluation of impairments constitutes an essential first step in rehabilitation management of the patient. When the physician and therapists understand the nature of the impairments, they can provide specific targeted therapy to optimize the rehabilitation program.

Evaluation of neurological impairments in a stroke patient is an essential part of the initial diagnostic examination and of the rehabilitation assessment. Specific aims of evaluation of impairments in stroke patients are summarized in Table 2.

---

[1]Department of Physical Medicine and Rehabilitation, Loma Linda University, 11234 Anderson St., Loma Linda, CA 92354, USA

Table 1. Medical diagnosis versus rehabilitation diagnosis.

Medical diagnosis
    Pathology (e.g., infarction) → Neurological deficits (e.g., hemiplegia)
Rehabilitation diagnosis
    Impairments (e.g., hemiplegia) → Disability (e.g., inability to walk)

Table 2. Aims of impairment evaluation.

1. Initial clinical examination
    a. Purpose
    Determine the etiology, pathology, localization, and severity of the lesion.
    Assess comorbidities.
    Monitor the subsequent clinical course.
    b. Timing
    Immediate and daily during the acute phase.
2. Rehabilitation assessment
    a. Purpose
    Identify patients most likely to benefit from rehabilitation, i.e., prognostication.
    Identify clinical problems that will form the focus of the rehabilitation plan.
    Select appropriate setting for rehabilitation.
    Monitor patient progress during rehabilitation.
    Evaluate the outcome.
    b. Timing
    Immediately post acute (2–7 days post onset).
    Subsequent follow-up at appropriate intervals.

Initial Clinical Examination

The initial clinical examination of a patient with an acute stroke includes a thorough, detailed neurological examination. Identification of the specific neurological impairments helps the clinician establish the etiology, pathology, anatomical localization, and severity of the stroke. Measurement of neurological impairments in the acute phase of care of stroke patients is most often recorded in clinical descriptive terms. It is unusual for the clinician to use quantitative measures or scaled tests to define neurological impairments. Details of the customary clinical tests encompassed by the standard neurological examination may be found in standard textbooks, and these are not discussed in this chapter.

The initial assessment of the patient provides the clinician with the information needed to prescribe acute intervention and is the basis for subsequent decisions regarding rehabilitation [1]. Additional information about the patient's general medical status and presence of comorbidities is extremely important in planning for the ongoing care provided by the rehabilitation practitioner.

Rehabilitation Assessment

The initial assessment of a stroke patient for rehabilitation may be performed as soon as the patient is stable neurologically and medically. This could be as early as day 2 post onset. The advantages of early rehabilitation evaluation are that conclusions can often be made in the acute phase about prognosis and suitability for rehabilitation. Once the patient has been evaluated, specific therapy can be initiated promptly.

The nature of the impairments observed in the first several days may, however, be distorted by the evolving physiological and pathological changes in the brain. For example, severe impairments noted on day 2 may be much less severe on day 7. Thus, it is customary to base predictions about recovery on clinical observations made 6–7 days post onset rather than day 2 or 3.

Assessment of the patient's general medical status and coimpairments are very important for decisions regarding rehabilitation. Important conditions impacting the management of the patient are cardiovascular diseases (hypertension, ischemic heart disease, congestive cardiac failure, arrhythmia), diabetes mellitus, chronic pulmonary diseases (asthma, chronic bronchitis, emphysema), locomotor disorders (amputation, arthritis), psychiatric disease, and other neurological diseases (Parkinson's, Alzheimer's). The remainder of this chapter addresses only issues relating to neurological impairment.

Assessment of Neurological Impairments

A detailed list of neurological impairments encountered in post acute stroke patients is described under the following headings: higher mental function, language, cranial nerves, motor system, sensory system, and posture and balance.

Higher Mental Function

Focal brain lesions associated with a stroke frequently produce measurable impairments in higher mental function. Even small lesions may significantly impair cognition, particularly when there are multiple focal lesions. However, interpretation of test information must be made in the context of the clinical situation because other nonstroke factors may contribute to impaired mental status. Many patients are elderly and may have had some premorbid decline in mental status. Further, general medical disorders such as a fever, electrolyte disturbance, hypothyroidism, congestive heart failure, and reaction to medication may produce an encephalopathy. Such patients are often confused and may have a diminished level of consciousness; they have a generalized disturbance of mental status with abnormalities in most or all cognitive tests. The encephalopathy associated with these general medical problems is reversible following correction of the complicating disorder. It is only after nonstroke factors have been excluded that changes in mental status can be attributed to the focal lesion of the brain.

The cognitive impairments observed with focal lesions frequently show specific disturbances, for example, memory loss, neglect, or constructional apraxia. Disturbances such as these can usually be recognized at the bedside. Because cognitive impairments can have a significant influence on the rehabilitation program and on outcome, the bedside mental status examination should be an essential part of the assessment of every stroke patient. The components of the examination are shown in Table 3. For a detailed description of the components of this assessment, see Strub and Black [2].

The Mini-Mental State Examination developed by Folstein et al. [3] is a useful bedside tool that screens a variety of mental domains quickly and gives a well-

Table 3. Mental status examination.

Level of consciousness
  Alertness, response to stimulation
Attention
Memory
  Orientation, new learning, remote memory
Cognition
  Fund of knowledge, calculation, problem solving, abstract thinking, judgment
Perception, apraxia, constructional ability
Affect and behavior

validated measure of overall mental function. In particular, it reflects memory, attention, orientation, language, and calculation. It requires fewer than 10 min to administer. Formal psychological tests may be used to establish global intellectual level and to reveal specific areas of diminished performance reflecting focal brain impairment. The Weschler Adult Intelligence Scale (WAIS) is commonly used in stroke patients.

Perceptual impairments are extremely important in stroke rehabilitation, and their recognition is an essential part of the higher mental function evaluation. A perceptual deficit is an impairment in the recognition and interpretation of sensory information when the sensory input system is intact, and is caused by a lesion at the cortical level. The term "neglect" is often used to describe selective inattention, which can often be detected by carefully observing the behavior of the patient. Unilateral neglect may be visual, tactile, spatial, or auditory. Visual neglect is demonstrated when the patient, on request, attempts to draw numbers on a clock face, draw a stick figure, or to bisect a horizontal line on a piece of paper. The patient is inattentive to the affected side. A patient who ignores the affected side because of a homonymous hemianopia does so because of impaired sensory input and hence does not have true neglect.

The term apraxia describes the inability of a patient to execute a willed movement when motor and sensory function are apparently preserved. Apraxia may be detected when a patient is unable to carry out a task on command such as "comb your hair" or "wave goodbye" even though there is no paralysis.

Communication Disorders

Communication is a complex function involving reception, central processing, and sending of information. Communication occurs through the use of language and consists of a system of symbols that are combined to convey ideas, that is, letters, words, or gestures. Impairment of language is called aphasia, and its presence reflects an abnormality in the dominant hemisphere [4].

Speech is a term that refers to the motor mechanisms involved in the production of spoken words, namely breathing, phonation, and articulation. Dysphonia and dysarthria are disorders of speech.

Aphasia

Although there are many classification schemes for aphasia, certain identifiable groups of patients are observed with clinically similar disorders of communication.

Categorization of aphasia in a patient with stroke is important in clinical management because it provides a basis for predicting language recovery and also forms the basis for specific therapeutic intervention.

In the simplest classification, aphasia is divided into two main categories: motor aphasia (sometimes called expressive or anterior aphasia), characterized by nonfluent speech, and sensory aphasia, (sometimes called receptive, posterior, or Wernicke's aphasia), characterized by fluent speech. Eight categories of aphasia are listed in Table 4.

Use of simple bedside tests can allow the clinician to categorize the communication disorder according to the classification in Table 4. During informal clinical evaluation, the clinician should avoid using nonverbal cues such as gestures.

The following questions are addressed during the bedside assessment of aphasia:

Question	Clinical test
Does the patient understand?	Give verbal commands, ask patient to point to objects.
Is the patient able to talk?	Ask the patient to name objects, describe them, count. Listen for spontaneous speech.
Can the patient repeat?	Ask the patient to repeat words.
Can the patient read?	Give commands in writing.
Can the patient write?	Ask patient to copy or to write dictated words.

Complete evaluations of patients can be performed using formal aphasia tests. The following list summarizes the more commonly used formal aphasia tests:

1. The Boston Diagnostic Aphasia Examination [5] produces a classification of the aphasic features observed in a particular patient. It is also scored so that the severity of the aphasia can be compared to aphasic patients in general.
2. The Western Aphasia Battery [6] is somewhat similar to the Boston. It measures various parameters of spontaneous speech and examines comprehension, fluency, object naming, and repetition. It provides a total score called an aphasia quotient, which is a measure of the severity of the aphasia.
3. The Porch Index of Communication Ability (PICA) is different from the other tests in that it evaluates verbal, gestural, and graphic responses. It is very structures in its format and must be given by a trained professional. It provides a useful statistical summary of the details of the language impairments.

Table 4. Classification of aphasia.

Classification	Fluency	Comprehension	Repetition	Naming
Global	Poor	Poor	Poor	Poor
Brocas	Poor	Good	Variable	Poor
Isolation	Poor	Poor	Good	Poor
Transcortical motor	Poor	Good	Good	Poor
Wernicke's	Good	Poor	Poor	Poor
Transcortical sensory	Good	Poor	Good	Poor
Conduction	Good	Good	Poor	Poor
Anomic	Good	Good	Good	Poor

4. The Functional Communication Profile [7] provides an overall rating of functional communication. It is not a diagnostic test. The score indicates severity and can be a useful indicator of recovery.

For assessment of dysarthria, clinicians subjectively rate the degree of impairment as a percent intelligibility of speech.

Cranial Nerves

In patients with lesions involving the hemispheres, visual field defects may be present. Patients with hemianopia will often fail to detect objects on the affected side of the body, conferring significant disability. The defect can be characterized by confrontation testing.

Dysphagia may occur with unilateral hemisphere stroke, but it is much more pronounced in bilateral disease and in brainstem lesions. Lesions of the pons and medulla can produce a large variety of cranial nerve dysfunctions. No attempt is made to describe these in this chapter; the reader is referred to standard neurological texts.

Motor Impairment

Paralysis is such a common feature among central nervous system (CNS) impairments with stroke referred for rehabilitation that the terms hemiplegia and stroke are often used interchangeably. Assessment of motor impairment includes evaluation of tone, strength, coordination, and balance.

Strength

The most widely used scale to assess strength is the Medical Research Council (MRC) 6-point scale of 0 to 5 in which 0 represents complete paralysis, 3 is the ability to fully move the joint against gravity, and 5 indicates normal strength. The test is insensitive in its upper range. It is most useful in grading strength in patients with lower motor neuron lesions. The MRC scale is designed to assess the strength of individual muscles.

There are drawbacks in using this scale in upper motor neuron lesions such as stroke. A patient recovering from hemiplegia may not be able to selectively activate a particular muscle in isolation and hence would be given a 0 grade on the MRC scale, but may well be able to forcefully activate the muscle within a gross movement pattern in which groups of muscles contract together in synergy, for example, a flexor or extensor synergy pattern. Further, as tone increases during recovery, the capacity of the patient to move a joint may be restricted by spasticity in the antagonists. Cocontraction of agonists and antagonists can diminish the force of muscle contraction recorded externally. For example, assessment of strength in the wrist and finger extensors of a hemiparetic upper limb is quite difficult if the forearm flexors are spastic.

Despite these shortcomings, the MRC scale may be quite useful in the early phases following a stroke before significant spasticity develops. Demeunisse et al. [8] modified the MRC scale and developed a composite measure called the Motoricity Index in which three movements in the arm and three movements in the leg are rated and the

Table 5. The motoricity index (from [8 with permission]).

Test	Movement
1	Pinch grip—1-in. cube between thumb and index finger
2	Elbow flexion
3	Shoulder abduction
4	Ankle dorsiflexion
5	Knee extension
6	Hip flexion

Test	Score	Criterion
1	00	No movement
	33	Beginning of prehension
	56	Cube gripped, but not antigravity
	65	Holds cube against gravity
	77	Holds cube against resistance, but weak
	100	Normal
2–6	00	No movement
	28	Palpable contraction, but no movement
	42	Movement without gravity
	56	Movement against gravity
	74	Movement against resistance, but weak
	100	Normal

Arm score = (Scores of $1 + 2 + 3$)/3
Leg score = (Scores of $4 + 5 + 6$)/3
Total score = (Arm + leg)/2

Table 6. Brunnstrom stages of motor recovery (from [10 with permission]).

Stage	Characteristics
Stage 1	No activation of the limb.
Stage 2	Spasticity appears, and weak basic flexor and extensor synergies are present.
Stage 3	Spasticity is prominent. The patient voluntarily moves the limb, but muscle activation is all with the synergy patterns.
Stage 4	The patient begins to activate muscles selectively outside the flexor and extensor synergies.
Stage 5	Spasticity decreases, most muscle activation is selective and independent from the limb synergies.
Stage 6	Isolated movements are performed in a smooth, phasic, well-coordinated manner.

results combined into a total score. Details of the rating are shown in Table 5. The usefulness of the notoricity index is enhanced by the addition of a scale for trunk control developed by Sheikh et al. [9]. The trunk control scale was part of a larger assessment of motor function.

Brunnstrom [10] adopted a different approach for assessment of motor function in hemiparetic patients; she developed a test in which movement patterns are evaluated and motor function is rated according to stages of motor recovery. The clinician assesses the presence of flexor and extensor synergies and the degree of selective muscle activation from the synergy pattern (Table 6). The rating can be performed very quickly, and although the scale only defines recovery in broad categories, these categories do correlate with progressive functional recovery [11].

Table 7. Modified Ashworth scale (from [15 with permission]).

Grade	Description
0	No increase in muscle tone.
1	Slight increase in muscle tone, minimal resistance at the end of range of motion, catch and release.
2	Slight increase in muscle tone, manifested by a Catch, followed by minimal resistance through the remainder (less than half) of the range of motion.
3	More marked increase in muscle tone through most of range of motion, but affected part is easily moved.
4	Considerable increase in muscle tone; passive movement difficult.
5	Affected part rigid in flexion or extension.

Rather than subjectively assess strength using the MRC scale, Bohannon advocated direct measurement of force with a dynamometer [12]. Despite the limitations of assessing and interpreting muscle strength in patients with upper motor neuron lesions, strength does correlate with performance on functional tasks [13]. Fugl-Meyer et al. [14] designed a more detailed and comprehensive motor scale in which 50 different movements and abilities were rated. The test evaluates strength, reflexes, and coordination, and a composite score is derived on a scale of 0 to 100. The Fugl-Meyer scale is reliable, and repeat scores reflect motor recovery over time. It is quite useful and informative but has not been widely adopted by clinicians because it is time-consuming to complete each evaluation.

Tone

Muscle tone refers to the resistance felt when the examiner passively stretches a muscle by moving a joint. The rating is subjective and depends on the judgment of the examiner. Physiological conditions such as position of body segments strongly influence the level of muscle tone, and these must be controlled for as much as possible. The posture of the body greatly affects muscle tone. Tone will be increased if the patient is supine rather than prone, or standing rather than sitting. A high level of anxiety will also increase the degree of muscle tone.

Spasticity refers to a neurophysiological state of increased activity in the myotatic reflex that is reflected in increased resistance of a muscle when it is passively stretched. Quantitation of spasticity is difficult. The most widely used scale is the Ashworth Scale (Table 7) [15]. This scale is reliable and has proven useful as an outcome measure in clinical trials of treatment of spasticity.

Sensory Impairment

When sensory deficits exist as part of a clinical picture following a stroke, they frequently accompany motor impairment in the same anatomical distribution. Interpretation of sensory testing may be difficult in a confused or cognitively impaired patient. Clinical examination involves testing pain, temperature, touch, joint position, kinesthesia, and vibration. Lesions of the thalamus may cause severe contralateral sensory loss. With lesions in the cortex, sensation, although preserved, is qualitatively and quantitatively reduced. Parietal lobe lesions cause perceptual deficits as described earlier.

Balance, Coordination, and Posture

Impaired balance may be caused by deficits in motor and sensory function, by cerebellar lesions, and through vestibular dysfunction. Clinical testing involves assessing coordination using finger-to-nose pointing and alternating movements.

The ability of the patient to sit unsupported or, if able, to stand and walk provides important information. Ataxia caused by sensory impairment can be differentiated from ataxia from cerebellar loss because performance of a motor task with the eyes closed is much poorer in sensory ataxia.

Balance can be scored using the Berg Balance Assessment [16], which measures a number of separate items relating to balance. It is a simple test that can be completed in less than 10 min.

Evaluation of the neurological impairments should be made repeatedly during the course of the rehabilitation program. Ideally, evaluations should be made weekly in the early phases of rehabilitation, to allow monitoring of the recovery process and to guide the therapeutic intervention.

In addition to defining the neurological impairments associated with the stroke, the rehabilitation team is concurrently interested in loss of function, that is, disability. As rehabilitation proceeds, functional assessment of activities of daily living, mobility, etc., progressively becomes the principal focus of ongoing evaluation.

Comorbidities and Coimpairments

A stroke patient may have any of numerous other medical disorders, called comorbidities. Some examples of comorbidities are heart disease, chronic obstructive lung disease, peripheral vascular disease, diabetes mellitus, other neurological disorders such as Parkinson's disease, polyneuropathy, and arthritis. These disorders, when present, will confer additional limitations on the patient's functional status. These limitations are often referred to as coimpairments. Some examples of coimpairments are joint pain and deformity from arthritis, angina, decreased effort tolerance, limb ischemia, amputation, and sensory loss from polyneuropathy. The rehabilitation team should carefully assess all these factors as a prelude to judging the functional prognosis, determining the ability of the patient to actively participate in the rehabilitation program, and defining the specifics of the rehabilitation program.

References

1. Wade DT, Langton Hewer R, Skillbeck CE, David RM (1985) Stroke: a critical approach to diagnosis, treatment and management. Year Book, Chicago
2. Strub R, Black F (1985) The mental status examination in neurology, 2nd edn. Davis, Philadelphia
3. Folstein MF, Folstein SF, McHugh PR (1975) Mini-mental state: a practical method for grading the cognitive state of patients for the clinician. J Psychiatr Res 12:189–198
4. Kertesz A (1987) Communication disorders. In: Brandstater ME, Basmajian J (eds) Stroke rehabilitation. Williams and Wilkins, Baltimore, pp 283–305
5. Goodglass H, Kaplan E (1984) Boston diagnostic aphasia examination (BDAE). Lea and Febiger, Philadelphia
6. Kertesz A (1982) Western aphasia battery. Grune and Stratton, New York

7. Sarno MT (1969) The functional communication profile: manual of directions. Rehabilitation monograph 42. Institute of Rehabilitation Medicine, New York
8. Demuerisse A, Demol O, Robaye E (1980) Motor evaluation in vascular hemiplegia. Eur Neurol 19:382–389
9. Sheikh K, Smith DS, Meade TW, Brennan PJ, Ide L (1980) Assessment of motor function in studies of chronic disability. Rheumatol Rehabil 19:83–90
10. Brunnstrom S (1970) Movement therapy in hemiplegia: a neuromuscular approach. Harper and Row, New York
11. Brandstater ME, deBruin H, Gowland C, Clarke B (1983) Hemiplegic gait: analysis of temporal variables. Arch Phys Med Rehabil 64:583–587
12. Bohannon RW (1989) Is the measurement of muscle strength appropriate in patients with brain lesions? Phys Ther 69:225–230
13. Bohannon RW (1989) Correlation of lower limb strengths and other variables with standing performance in stroke patients. Physiother Can 41:198–202
14. Fugl-Meyer AR, Jaasko L, Leyman I, Olsson S, Steglind S (1975) The post-stroke hemiplegic patient. I: A method for evaluation of physical performance. Scand J Rehab Med 7:13–31
15. Bohannon RW, Smith MB (1987) Interrater reliability of a modified Ashworth scale of muscle spasticity. Phys Ther 67:206–207
16. Berg K, Wood-Dauphinee S, Williams JI, Gayton D (1989) Measuring balance in the elderly: preliminary development of an instrument. Physiother Can 41:304–311

Stroke Impairment Assessment Set* (SIAS)

Naoichi Chino, Shigeru Sonoda, Kazuhisa Domen, Eiichi Saitoh, and Akio Kimura[1]

Summary. A new method for the evaluation of stroke patients, designated the Stroke Impairment Assessment Set (SIAS), is presented. The SIAS primarily employs single-task assessment of various functions and rates performance on scales of 0 to 5 or 0 to 3. The items evaluated include motor function, muscle tone, sensation, range of motion, pain, trunk control, visuospatial perception, aphasia, and function on the unaffected side. Scores for each item are plotted on a radar chart so that deficits can be identified at a glance. The interobserver variation in SIAS scores is acceptable, and assessment can be performed as part of a routine clinical examination.

Introduction

Survivors of stroke continue to increase in number. This is particularly so in Japan, and a recent survey by the Ministry of Health and Welfare indicated that about 43% of patients aged 65 years or older who were institutionalized for at least 6 months had suffered a stroke [1].

There is no doubt that we as physiatrists must develop new methods or improve our traditional modalities to enable these patients to return to life in their own community. To carry out effective rehabilitation of stroke patients, we initially need to make an accurate evaluation of the level of impairment [2]. Thus, a more scientific regimen is required in rehabilitation medicine, and the evaluation and treatment of impairment must be given more attention than the care of disability.

Wade et al. [3,4] have introduced a method that primarily evaluates arm function as well as the other parts of the body, and Fugl-Meyer et al. [5] provided a method for the evaluation of physical performance in poststroke hemiplegic patients. However, these methods require either sophisticated equipment that is not generally available or the knowledge of reflexes which are not assessed during routine physical examination.

We recently developed a new evaluation method for stroke patients called the Stroke Impairment Assessment Set (SIAS), and we have found it can be used to evaluate various aspects of impairment in hemiplegics, including motor, sensory, and motion impairment, as well as other deficits. We adopted some of the items in our

[1]Department of Rehabilitation Medicine, Keio University School of Medicine, 35 Shinanamachi, Shinjuku-ku, Tokyo 160, Japan
* Reprinted with some modifications from the Jpn J Rehabil Med 31:119–125, 1994

original SIAS from the Symposium on Methodologic Issues in Stroke Outcome Research [6] conducted by Gresham, Granger, and Basmajian (in Buffalo, NY, USA, July 1989).

This chapter presents an outline of the SIAS so that not only the physiatrist but also other health care professionals will be encouraged to improve the evaluation and treatment of stroke patients by focusing on impairment.

Methods

A functional assessment and rehabilitation regimen should be carefully devised for each patient on the basis of the International Classification of Impairments, Disabilities and Handicaps (ICIDH), which was developed by the World Health Organization (WHO) in 1980 [2].

When evaluating the impairment of a stroke patient, the major items that should be covered are as listed in Table 1. The SIAS primarily involves single-task assessment of various functions and rates the patient's performance on a scale (usually 0–5 or 0–3). The total SIAS score range is from 0 (total impairment) to 76 (normal function).

Motor Function of the Upper Extremity

The upper and lower extremities are evaluated separately, and proximal and distal function is also examined separately.

In the upper extremity, the knee-mouth test is designed to evaluate proximal function, and the finger test is used for distal function. If a patient is able to touch the

Table 1. Stroke impairment assessment set (SIAS).

	U/E	L/E
Motor function		
Proximal	0–5	0–5 (hip)
		0–5 (knee)
Distal	0–5	0–5
Tone		
DTRs	0–3	0–3
Muscle tone	0–3	0–3
Sensory function		
Touch	0–3	0–3
Position	0–3	0–3
ROM	0–3	0–3
Pain	0–3	
Trunk balance	0–3 (abdominal MMT)	
	0–3 (verticality test)	
Visuospatial	0–3	
Speech	0–3	
Unaffected side	0–3	0–3
Total score:	76	

UE, upper extremity; L/E, lower extremity; ROM, range of motion; DTR, deep tendon reflexes; MMT, manual muscle testing.

Fig. 1. Knee mouth

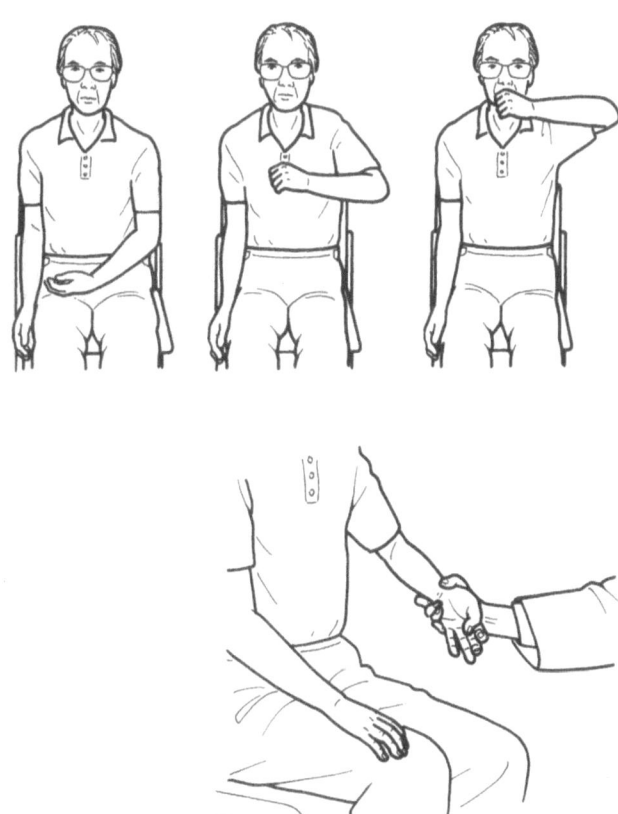

Fig. 2. Finger function

contralateral knee with the affected hand and bring it back to the mouth, a score of 3 is given. A score of 5 indicates that the patient carries out the knee-mouth test as smoothly as on the unaffected side. When the patient can only lift the hand to the level of the nipple, a score of 2 is given. If no muscle contraction is noted in the biceps brachii, a score of 0 is given (Fig. 1).

Individual finger movements are tested to assess distal function. If the patient can adequately flex and extend each digit, a score of 3 is given, while a score of 5 indicates normal coordination. A score of 2 means that the patient can move each finger but is unable to extend and flex them completely. A score of 1 is given for gross finger flexion or mass movement, and 0 is assigned for a complete lack of voluntary finger movement (Fig. 2).

Motor Function of the Lower Extremity

In evaluating the lower extremity, proximal motor function is tested by hip flexion in the sitting position. A score of 5 indicates that the patient can flex the affected hip joint as smoothly as on the unaffected side. A score of 3 means the patient can flex the hip so that the foot is completely off the floor, while a score of 2 is given if the foot is barely lifted off the floor. A score of 0 means that no voluntary hip flexion is noted (Fig. 3).

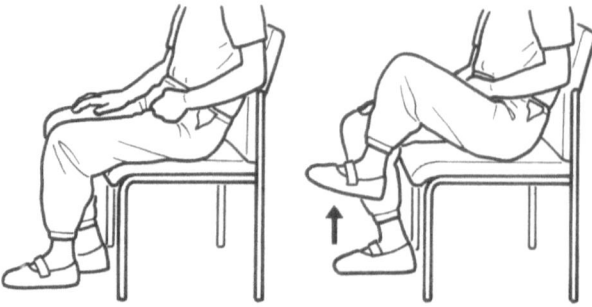

Fig. 3. Hip flexion

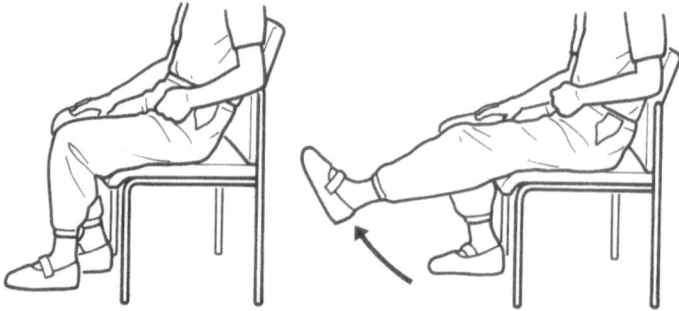

Fig. 4. Knee extension

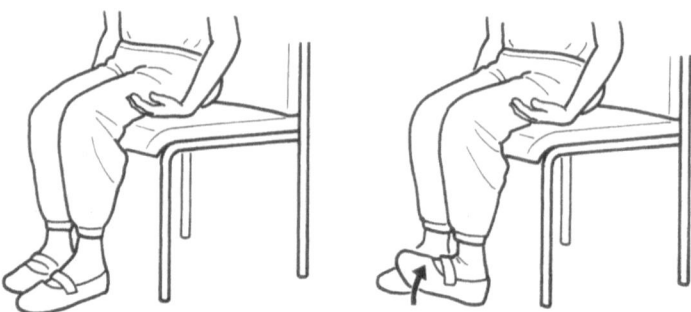

Fig. 5. Foot tap

The knee extension test is also used to assess proximal motor function in the lower extremity. When the patient is able to extend the knee joint with same strength and repetition as those of the unaffected side, a score of 5 is given. When the knee joint can be extended against gravity and with some clumsiness, a score of 3 is assigned (Fig. 4). If the patient can contract the knee extensors and lift the heel off the floor but is unable to extend the knee joint fully, a score of 2 is given. A score of 0 means no contraction of the quadriceps muscles occurs.

Ankle dorsiflexion with the foot on the floor is examined to assess distal motor function. If the patient is able to dorsiflex the ankle and lift the front of the foot away from the floor, a score of 3 is given. A score of 5 signifies normal muscle strength and foot-tap coordination (Fig. 5). If the tibialis anterior muscle shows no contraction, then the score is 0. Scores of 4 and 2 are assigned for the intervening levels of ability.

When the patient is unable to sit up in a chair because of acute stroke or poor balance, we use manual muscle testing [7] and estimate the functional score.

Tone

Muscle tone is evaluated by using both the deep tendon reflexes and the passive joint resistance of the upper and lower extremities. Deep tendon reflexes (DTRs) are graded as follows: a score of 0 indicates that reflexes (e.g., the biceps and triceps reflexes in the upper limbs and the patellar and Achilles' tendon reflexes in the lower limbs) are all markedly increased and that even finger flexor clonus or ankle clonus is present. When the tendon reflexes are moderately increased, a score of 2 is given. A score of 1 means that these reflexes are slightly exaggerated or are absent. A score of 3 signifies normal or symmetrical reflexes when compared to the unaffected side (Figs. 6 and 7).

To assess muscle tone, a score of 0 is given when the tone is remarkably increased by passive motion. If muscle tone is moderately increased, a score of 1 is given, and the same score applies when tone is diminished. A score of 2 indicates that muscle tone is only slightly increased, while a score of 3 means that the tone is normal (Figs. 8 and 9).

Sensory Function

Light touch sensation is checked on the palm of the hand and the dorsum of the foot. A score of 0 means anesthesia and a score of 3 is normal, with evaluation being based on the examiner's clinical judgment (Fig. 10). To assess position sense, we use the index finger or thumb in the upper extremity and the great toe in the lower extremity. When no position change is detected by the patient after the maximum possible motion, a score of 0 is given. A score of 1 means that the patient recognizes movement

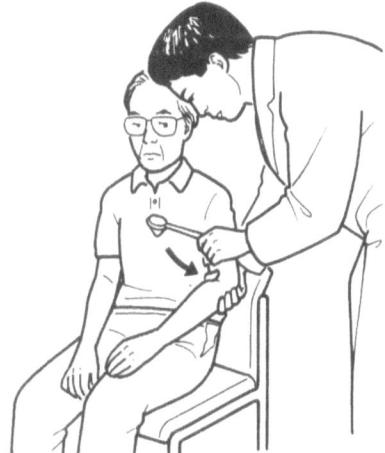

Fig. 6. DTR U/E

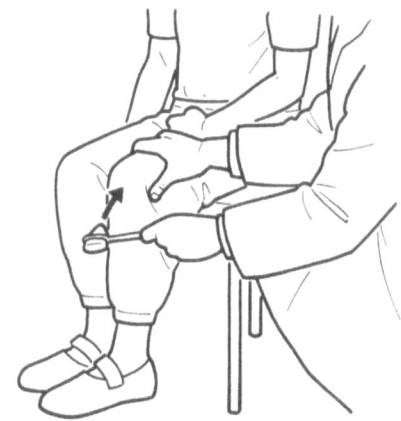

Fig. 7. DTR L/E

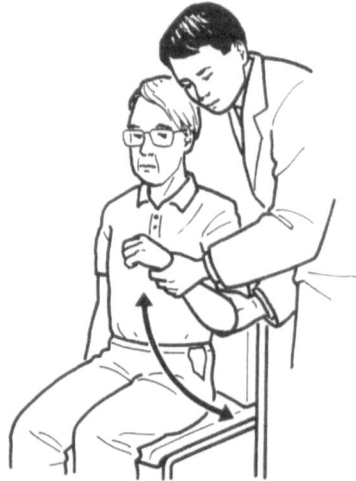

Fig. 8. Tone   U/E

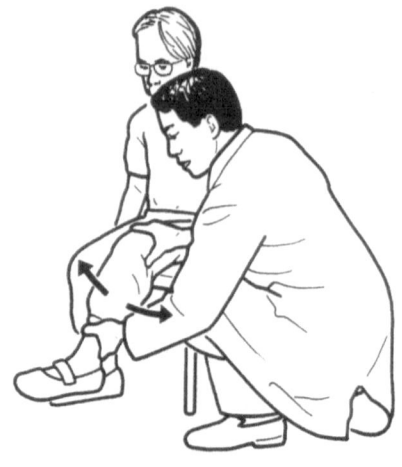

Fig. 9. Tone   L/E

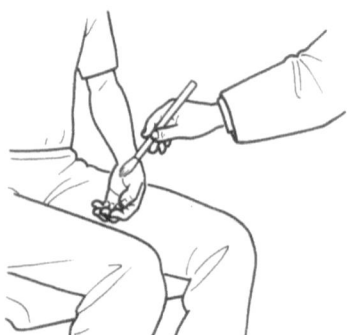

Fig. 10. Superficial   U/E

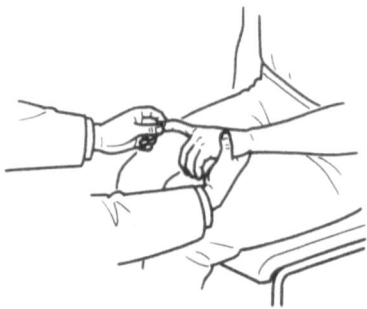

Fig. 11. Position   U/E

of the digits but not the correct direction, even at maximal excursion. When the patient can correctly perceive the direction of a moderate excursion, the score is 2. A score of 3 means that the patient can correctly identify the direction of a slight movement (Figs. 11 and 12).

Range of Motion

Because the shoulder and the ankle are the major joints that most readily develop contractures, these are the target joints to be examined for range of motion (ROM).

When passive shoulder abduction is limited to less than 45° (normally 180°), a score of 0 is given. A score of 1 means that the joint can be abducted from 45° to 90°, and a score of 2 indicates abduction from 90° to 150°. A score of 3 indicates that abduction of the shoulder beyond 150° is possible (Fig. 13).

In the case of ankle dorsiflexion, a score of 0 means that passive dorsiflexion (with the knee fully extended) is limited to less than 10° of plantar flexion (−10° of

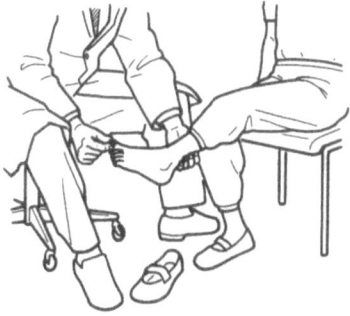

Fig. 12. Position L/E

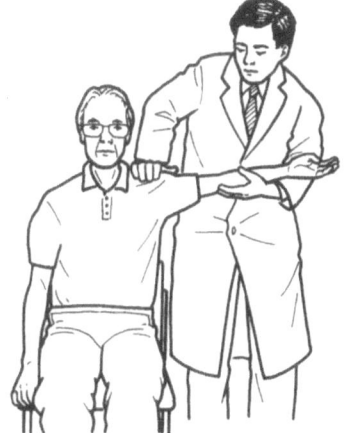

Fig. 13. Shoulder ROM

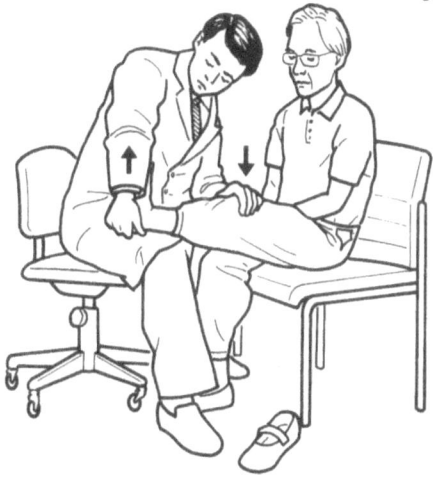

Fig. 14. Ankle ROM

dorsiflexion). When dorsiflexion of the ankle is limited to 0°, a score of 1 is allocated. If the ankle moves up from 0° to 10°, the score is graded as 2, and a score of 3 is given when ankle dorsiflexion exceeds 10° (Fig. 14).

Pain

A score of 0 means that pain is so severe that this interferes with sleep (pain usually affects the shoulder joints, fingers, or other major joints of the body, but this category also includes the thalamic or central pain syndrome). When pain is moderate and does not interfere with sleep, a score of 2 is given. A score of 3 indicates that the patient does not complain of pain. (Pain not arising from a stroke-related case, e.g., pain caused by degenerative arthritis or kidney stones, should be disregarded in this assessment.)

Trunk Control

To carry out the essential activities of daily living, head and trunk control are of vital importance. Our preliminary study has indicated that head and trunk control are closely correlated with abdominal muscle strength. Vertical balance is also an important element of trunk control, so we evaluate this item in two categories.

First, we evaluate abdominal muscle strength as follows: the patient rests in the 45° semireclining position in a wheelchair or high-back chair and is asked to raise the shoulders off the back of the chair and assume a sitting position. If the patient is unable to sit up, the score is 0. A score of 1 indicates that the patient can sit up provided there is no resistance to the movement. If the patient can come to the sitting position despite pressure on the sternum by the examiner, a score of 2 is given. A score of 3 means that the patient has good strength in the abdominal muscles and is able to sit up against considerable resistance (Fig. 15).

Second, in the verticality test, a score of 0 is given if the patient can not maintain a sitting position. When a sitting position can only be maintained while tilting to one side and the patient is unable to correct the posture to the erect position, this is scored as 1. A score of 2 indicates that the patient can sit vertically when reminded to do so. If the patient can sit vertically in a normal manner, this is scored as 3 (Fig. 16). If the patient is not allowed to assume the upright position because of medical complications, such as an acute posthemorrhagic stage, impairment of consciousness, or hypotension, a score of 0 is also given.

Visuospatial Perception

A 50 cm-long tape measure is used and the central pointing method is adopted. The patient is asked to touch (with the unaffected thumb and index finger) the midportion of a tape held horizontally in front of himself or herself at a distance of about 50 cm. Two trials are allowed, and the largest error is used for scoring. If there is more than a 15-cm deviation from the central point, the score is 0. An error between 15 and 5 cm is scored as 1, a score of 2 indicates an error between 5 and 2 cm, and a score of 3 means deviation from the midpoint by less than 2 cm (Fig. 17).

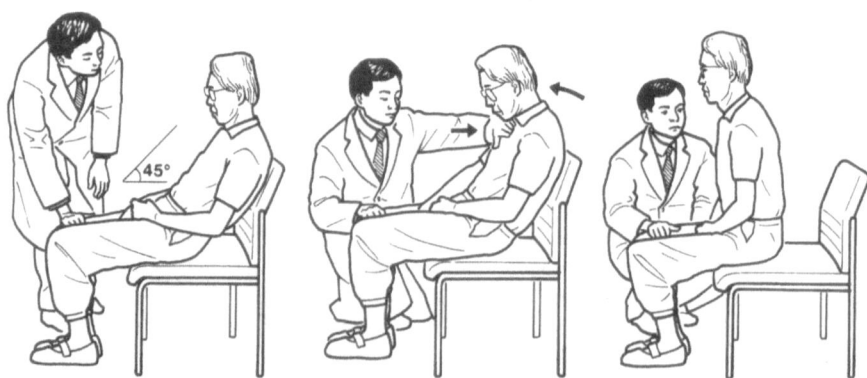

Fig. 15. Abdominal

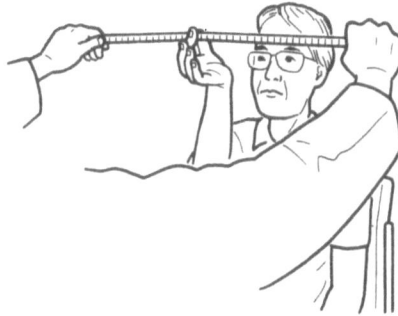

Fig. 17. Tape

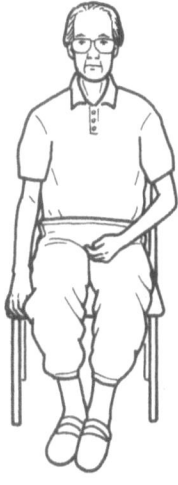

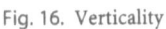

Fig. 16. Verticality

Aphasia

Both expression and comprehension are evaluated. A score of 0 means that the patient has total or global aphasia. If the patient is moderately or slightly aphasic, a score of 1 or 2, respectively, is given. A score of 3 means that there is no evidence of aphasia.

Function of the Unaffected Side

The hemiplegic side is always compared with the unaffected side, so the presence or absence of impairment on this side must also be evaluated. Such impairment may be caused by physiological aging or a premorbid condition.

The strength of the quadriceps muscle of the lower extremity and the grip strength of the upper extremity are determined. A score of 0 indicates severe quadriceps weakness relative to the patient's age (about antigravity strength). If the patient has moderate (grade 4 of the manual muscle testing [MMT] score) or minimal quadriceps weakness, a score of 1 or 2, respectively, is given. A score of 3 means normal strength (Fig. 18).

Our preliminary study indicated that a normal grip strength is greater than 25 kg for both men and women. Therefore, if the grip strength is above this level in two trials, a score of 3 is given. A score of 2 means a strength of 10–25 kg, and a score of 1 is given if a grip strength is 3–10 kg. If the grip strength is less than 3 kg, a score of 0 is given (Fig. 19).

Interobserver Variability of the SIAS

To examine the interobserver variability of the SIAS, two assessors (E.S. and S.S.) used the test to rate 12 stroke patients (10 men and 2 women aged 52–69 years; mean, 59 years). Six patients had ischemic stroke and the other 6 had hemorrhagic brain lesions.

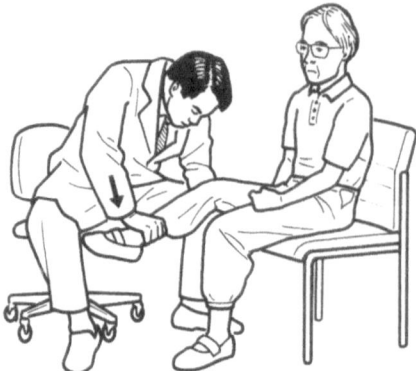

Fig. 18. Unaffected quadriceps

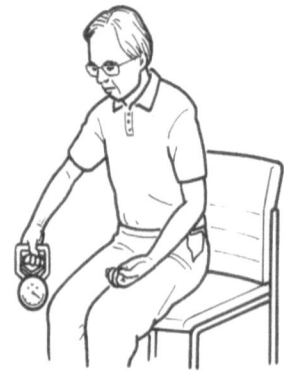

Fig. 19. Unaffected grip

Table 2. Interobserver variability of the SIAS: degree of agreement by weighted kappa ($n = 12$).

	U/E		L/E
Motor function			
Proximal	1.000		0.901 (hip)
			0.855 (knee)
Distal	0.976		0.891
Tone			
DTRs	0.625		0.615
Muscle tone	0.520		0.488
Sensory function			
Touch	0.500		0.500
Position	0.474		0.838
ROM	0.643		0.870
Pain		0.538	
Trunk balance			
Abdominal MMT		0.933	
Verticality test		0.625	
Visuospatial		0.776	
Speech		1.000	
Unaffected side	0.636		0.111

Interobserver variability was assessed using weighted-kappa statistical analysis [8]. As shown in Table 2, the scores for 9 of 22 items related to motor and communication function ranged from 0.838 to 1.000, and the correlation was very high. Scores for 6 items related to tendon reflexes and visuospatial function ranged from 0.615 to 0.776, and there was substantial interobserver agreement. Another 6 items related to pain and sensory function showed moderate agreement, with scores from 0.474 to 0.538. The remaining item (quadriceps strength on the unaffected side) showed poor correspondence (score, 0.111). However, all patients in this study were scored as either 2 or 3 for quadriceps strength and none were graded as 0 or 1. In this case, the analysis indicated only poor reliability [9] although the percentile correspondence of this item was fairly high, 66%.

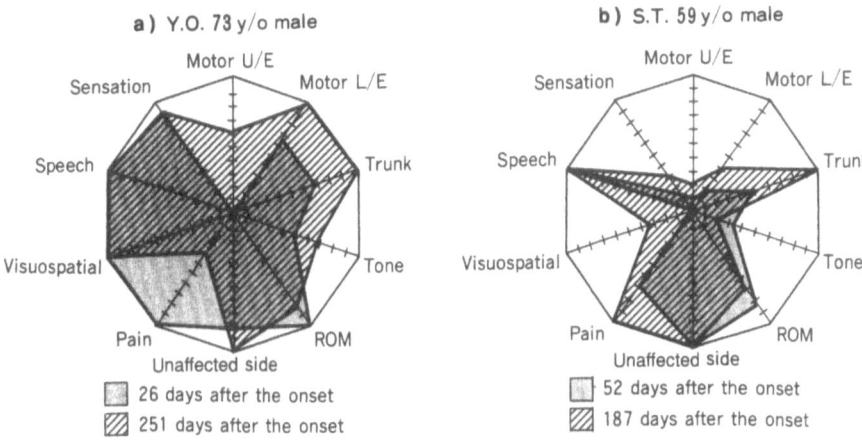

a) Y.O. 73 y/o male

b) S.T. 59 y/o male

26 days after the onset
251 days after the onset

52 days after the onset
187 days after the onset

Fig. 20. SIAS Radar Chart

Radar Charting System

Another feature of the SIAS is our method of recording the impairment of stroke patients. Scores for each item are plotted on a radar chart so that one can identify at a glance which areas of function are impaired or normal.

Figure 20a displays a SIAS radar chart for a 73-year-old man who suffered cerebral infarction 26 days before testing. This patient had severe impairment of motor function in the upper extremity and moderate impairment of the lower extremity. He also had moderate weakness of the upper and lower extremities on the unaffected side. His remaining functions were well preserved, and at the time of evaluation, he did not complain of pain. In the follow-up examination at 251 days after the onset of stroke, the motor function had improved from zero to moderate and there was complete recovery of the lower extremity. His trunk muscles and the sound side of the body had also recovered fully. However, he had developed some contractures of the extremities and moderate shoulder pain despite undergoing a rehabilitation program.

Figure 20b shows a radar chart for a 59-year-old man who had a cerebrovascular accident 52 days before this evaluation was made. His impairment was so severe on the affected side that only speech, ROM, and function on the sound side were preserved.

At the second SIAS evaluation 187 days after the ictus, he showed some recovery of his visuospatial deficit and reasonable trunk control. However, severe paralysis of his upper and lower extremities persisted and there was a severe sensory deficit. His ROM and muscle tone were somewhat worsened.

As shown by these examples, the patient's level of impairment can be followed during a rehabilitation program and the areas and extent of improvement can be easily determined. It is not necessary to plot all the items on the radar chart. Each clinician has a routine check-up system for stroke patients and can select the appropriate elements of the SIAS according to this system. However, it is advisable to plot the radar chart in the order of recording so that one can properly recognize deficits by reviewing the chart pattern.

Discussion

Since WHO established the ICIDH, it has become an international trend, particularly in the field of rehabilitation medicine, to evaluate dysfunction according to this system [2].

Many evaluation methods have been developed for chronically ill patients that focus on the level of disability and are related to the capacity for independent daily living [10], but hemiplegic patients can carry out most such activities of daily living with the unaffected extremity. Therefore, the functional evaluation of disability using such methods does not reflect the improvement of paralysis in stroke patients.

Brunnstrom [11] has advocated the assessment of motor recovery as a synergic pattern, but not all hemiplegic patients follow this process of recovery. Fugl-Meyer et al. [5] also used a motor recovery staging system similar to the Brunnstrom method along with assessment of other functions, such as pain, sensation, and ROM. However, the evaluation items are too numerous and the scoring system too vague for clinical use.

The Frenchay arm test [3] and the motoricity index [12] are designed to evaluate motor function on the basis of hand function or MMT. However, the hemiplegic patient behaves quite differently in motor testing when compared with patients who have peripheral nerve injuries. In addition, some evaluation methods employ sophisticated procedures and complicated grading systems and hence do not attract the interest of clinicians other than rehabilitation specialists.

The Canadian Neurological Scale [13] has recently been introduced and is designed to assess different levels of impairment in stroke patients. However, this system applies mainly to acute stroke patients and does not seem appropriate for assessment during rehabilitation.

The SIAS presented in this chapter is an evaluation procedure that can be carried out during an ordinary physical examination and can also be done by other medical professionals. To make evaluation simple, the SIAS uses single-task assessment to examine each item. Functional grading is done from 0 to 5 or 0 to 3 according to the traditional clinical scoring method, with the former scale being used for objective parameters such as motor function and the latter scale being used for subjective parameters such as pain and cognition.

Because the stroke patient undergoing rehabilitation will often be evaluated in the sitting position, the SIAS is designed for examining a patient seated in a wheelchair or in the reclining position and thus is widely applicable. Some examples are the items related to trunk control and abdominal muscle strength. Furthermore, it is accepted that the testing of communication skills and cognitive ability is more accurately performed with the patient in the sitting position rather than lying in bed. However, if the patient is bedridden, the motor function portion of the SIAS can still be estimated by conventional MMT.

Statistical evaluation of the SIAS showed satisfactory interobserver agreement for most items, although assessment of the unaffected leg was rather variable, perhaps because of the weighted-kappa analysis that was used. This subject may require for further investigation. Radar charts of the level of impairment provide a visual method of detecting functional deficits as well as areas of improvement or deterioration at a glance. Neurological function will improve spontaneously as well as with therapy, but joint contractures or muscle power on the sound side may sometimes deteriorate over time. The radar chart sensitively reflects such changes of function during follow-up.

In conclusion, we believe that the SIAS may improve the assessment of impairment in stroke patients and thus lead to a better outcome of rehabilitation.

References

1. Patient Survey 1987 (1989) 1:p41 statistics and Information Department, Ministry of Health and Welfare, Japan (in Japanese)
2. World Health Organization (1980) International classification of impairments, disabilities and handicaps. WHO, Geneva
3. Wade DT, Langton-Hewer R, Wood VA, Skilbeck CE, Ismail HM (1983) The hemiplegic arm after stroke: measurement and recovery. J Neurol Neurosurg Psychiatry 46:521–524
4. Collin C, Wade D (1990) Assessing motor impairment after stroke: a pilot reliability study. J Neurol Neurosurg Psychiatry 53:576–579
5. Fugl-Meyer AR, Jaasko L, et al (1975) The post-stroke hemiplegic patient. 1. A method for evaluation of physical performance. Scand J Rehabil Med 7:13–31
6. Gresham GE (ed) (1990) Methodologic issues in stroke outcome research. Stroke 21(9)(suppl II)
7. Daniels L, Williams M, et al (1956) Muscle testing. Saunders, Philadelphia
8. Lyden PD, Lau GT (1991) A critical appraisal of stroke evaluation and rating scales. Stroke 22:1345–1352
9. Spitznagel EL, Helzer JE (1985) A proposed solution to the base rate problem in the kappa statistic. Arch Gen Psychiatry 42:725–728
10. Gresham GE, Labi MLC (1984) Functional assessment instruments currently available for documenting outcomes in rehabilitation medicine. In: Granger CV, Gresham GE (eds) Functional assessment in rehabilitation medicine. William and Wilkins, Baltimore, pp 65–85
11. Brunnstrom S (1970) Movement therapy in hemiplegia. Harper and Row
12. Demeurisse G, Demol O, et al (1980) Motor evaluation in vascular hemiplegia. Eur Neurol 19:382–389
13. Cote R, Battista RN, et al (1989) The Canadian neurological scale. Neurology 39:638–643

Evaluation of Motor Function in Stroke Patients Using the Stroke Impairment Assessment Set (SIAS)

Kazuhisa Domen, Shigeru Sonoda, Naoichi Chino, Eiichi Saitoh, and Akio Kimura[1]

Summary. We have developed the Stroke Impairment Assessment Set (SIAS) as a global measure of stroke impairment. This chapter reviews our recent research on motor function in stroke patients using the SIAS. The affected-side motor assessment items of the SIAS were found to be reliable and valid for evaluating hemiplegia by employing the concepts of both synergy and muscle strength. The motor SIAS score was strongly correlated with the Brunnstrom stage (Spearman's $r = .694-.939$) and the manual muscle testing score (Spearman's $r = .870-.958$). However, some dispersion was caused by differences in the definitions employed by these scales. A longitudinal study indicated that motor SIAS items were more sensitive for detecting motor recovery after stroke than the Brunnstrom stage or manual muscle testing. The recovery of motor function at discharge could be predicted by the SIAS depending on whether the score on admission was 0 (no voluntary movement) or 1 (minimal voluntary movement). A cross-sectional study showed that unaffected-side function was an important factor in relation to disability, while a longitudinal study demonstrated that unaffected-side function also improves during rehabilitation (grip strength was 23.51 kg on admission and 25.54 kg on discharge; $n = 75$, $P < .01$). Therefore, unaffected-side function should also be measured when assessing stroke impairment.

Introduction

Motor impairment in hemiplegic stroke patients is the most important factor influencing disability [1]. Although many stroke assessment methods have been developed [2,3], no method effectively addresses the parameters of synergy and muscle strength when measuring motor impairment, that is, a scale based on synergy cannot measure muscle strength, and one based on muscle strength cannot describe the pattern of movement. The motor assessment items of the Stroke Impairment Assessment Set (SIAS) [4] were designed taking this problem into consideration.

[1]Department of Rehabilitation Medicine, Keio University School of Medicine, 35 Shinanomachi, Shinjuku-ku, Tokyo 160, Japan

Another problem with previous stroke scales is that unaffected-side function has been ignored. Because we consider that the unaffected side is important for the functional independence of stroke patients, the SIAS also includes assessment of such function to provide a global evaluation of stroke.

This chapter reviews our recent research on motor function in stroke patients using the SIAS and also discusses the value of the motor assessment items of the SIAS (SIAS-motor, SIAS-M).

Basic Principles of the SIAS and SIAS-M

We have been developing the SIAS since 1990. The SIAS consists of nine categories, which are divided into 22 items to describe the various aspects of stroke impairment. Some items of the SIAS are based on the proposals made at the Symposium on Methodologic Issues in Stroke Outcome Research conducted by Gresham, Granger, and Basmajian in Buffalo in 1989 [5]. According to the symposium recommendations, we adopted a rating scale of 3 or 5 points for each item.

The basic principles of the SIAS are as follows. (1) It contains the minimum number of items required for the evaluation of stroke impairment; (2) it can be easily used by physicians in daily practice; and (3) each item can be evaluated by the performance of a single test (single-task assessment). Accordingly, the SIAS can be completed in less than 10 min without any special equipment. Furthermore, because most of the SIAS items are based on techniques of the traditional neurological examination, it can be used by a variety of medical professionals. (Further details of the SIAS are described in the chapter by Chino et al., this volume.)

Our recent research has shown that the SIAS is a reliable and valid instrument for assessing stroke impairment [1,6,7]. Use of the 3- or 5-point scale allows the detection of a small change in impairment. Therefore, the SIAS can be applied not only to cross-sectional studies but also to longitudinal studies on the improvement in impairment.

We have designed five tests to evaluate the proximal and distal function of the affected-side upper and lower extremities (Table 1). The proximal upper extremity (U/E) and proximal lower extremity (L/E) tests utilize synergic movement patterns for the task assigned in the SIAS-M, while the other tests are nonsynergic movement patterns. All the SIAS-M items are scored from 0 to 3 points on the basis of the degree of achievement of a task, as is done with manual muscle testing (MMT) [8]. A score of 0 means that no voluntary movement is noted. If the subject performs the task, 3 points are given. A score of 3, 4, or 5 is used to distinguish the degree of clumsiness and speed of the performance. This basic pattern is maintained through all the SIAS-M items, so the SIAS-M can be learned easily and can also be applied to patients showing an atypical pattern of recovery.

Comparison of the SIAS-M with Other Motor Assessment Scales

To study the concurrent validity of the SIAS motor assessment test [9], we correlated each item with those in two other motor assessment scales, the manual muscle testing (MMT) and the Brunnstrom stage [10]. The MMT was performed according to the Motricity Index method [11].

The subjects, 77 stroke patients (mean age, 61.2 years), included 43 with cerebral hemorrhage and 34 with cerebral infarction (right brain damage, 43, left brain damage, 34). The time from onset varied from 159 days to 270 months (median, 989 days). Every SIAS motor item was highly correlated with the other two motor assessment scales. Spearman's correlation coefficients ranged from .694 to .939 between the SIAS-M and Brunnstrom stage, and from .870 to .958 between the SIAS-M and the MMT (Fig. 1). These results indicate that the validity of the SIAS motor assessment test is satisfactory.

Table 1. Stroke Impairment Assessment Set (SIAS) affected-side motor assessment items (SIAS-motor, SIAS-M) and unaffected-side motor function items.

Affected-Side Function (SIAS-M)

Proximal upper extremity (KNEE - MOUTH TEST)

In the sitting position, the patient touches the contralateral knee with the affected hand and then lifts it to the mouth. When the hand reaches the mouth, the affected-side shoulder is abducted to 90°. Then the hand is returned to the knee. The test is performed 3 times. If contracture of the shoulder or elbow is present, the test is judged on the basis of movement within the range of motion.

0: No contraction of biceps brachii.
1: Minimal voluntary movement is noted, but the patient cannot raise the hand to the level of the nipple.
2: Synergic movement is noted in the shoulder and elbow joints, but the patient is not able to touch the mouth with the affected-side hand.
3: The patient carries out the task with severe or moderate clumsiness.
4: The patient carries out the task with mild clumsiness.
5: The patient carries out the task as smoothly as on the unaffected side.

Distal upper extremity (FINGER FUNCTION TEST)

Individual finger movements are tested. The patient flexes each digit from thumb to little finger in that order and then extends them from little finger to thumb.

0: No voluntary finger movement.
1: 1A; Minimal voluntary movement or mass flexion.
   1B; Mass extension.
   1C; Minimal individual movement.
2: Individual movement of each finger is possible, but flexion or extension is not complete.
3: Individual movement of each finger is possible with adequate flexion and extension of the digits. However, the patient carries out the task with severe or moderate clumsiness.
4: The patient carries out the task with mild clumsiness.
5: The patient carries out the task as smoothly as on the unaffected side.

Proximal lower extremity (hip) (HIP FLEXION TEST)

In the sitting position, the patient flexes the hip as much as possible and returns it to the original position. The test is performed 3 times. The assessor may assist the patient in maintaining the sitting position if necessary.

0: No voluntary movement is noted.
1: Minimal movement is noted, but the foot is not lifted off the floor.
2: The foot is barely lifted off the floor.
3-5: The same definitions as for the KNEE-MOUTH TEST.

Table 1. *Continued.*

Proximal lower extremity (knee) (KNEE EXTENSION TEST)

In the sitting position with knee flexion of 90°, the patient extends the knee as much as possible and returns it to the original position. Slight knee flexion (approximately 10°) is allowed at full extension. The test is performed 3 times. The assessor may assist the patient in maintaining the sitting position if necessary.

0: No voluntary movement is noted.
1: Minimal movement is noted, but the foot is not lifted off the floor.
2: The foot is barely lifted off the floor.
3–5: The same definitions as for the KNEE – MOUTH TEST.

Distal lower extremity (FOOT-PAT TEST)

In the sitting or supine position, the patient dorsiflexes the ankle while keeping the heel on the floor as much as possible and then returns it to the original position. The task is performed 3 times. Then it is repeated as fast as possible.

0: No contraction of tibialis anterior.
1: Minimal movement is noted, but front of the foot is not lifted off the floor.
2: Ankle dorsiflexion is noted, but is less than the range of motion.
3–5: The same definitions as for the KNEE – MOUTH TEST.

Unaffected-Side Function

Grip strength

In the sitting position with the elbow extended, the measured values (kg) are recorded. Preliminary scores are as follows.

0: <3 kg
1: 3–10 kg
2: 10–25 kg
3: >25 kg

Quadriceps muscle strength

In the sitting position, extension of the unaffected-side quadriceps is measured.

0: Severe quadriceps weakness (about antigravity strength or less)
1: Moderate quadriceps weakness (grade 4 of the manual muscle testing [MMT] score)
2: Minimal quadriceps weakness
3: Normal strength

The following characteristics of the SIAS-M were also demonstrated by our investigation:

1. Patients in a single Brunnstrom stage (e.g., U/E stage 3 or 5, or finger stage 5, or L/E stages 3, 4, and 5) were divided into three to five levels by the SIAS-M. This dispersion was caused by differences in the degree of clumsiness as defined by the SIAS-M in Brunnstrom stage 4 or 5 patients, and by the differences in achievement of the SIAS-M task against gravity in Brunnstrom stage 3 patients.

2. Patients with an MMT of 3 or more tended to be dispersed over two to four different levels by the SIAS-M. This dispersion was caused by differences in the degree of clumsiness as defined by the SIAS-M in patients with the same MMT level or by differences in the task used for evaluation (e.g., individual finger movements in the SIAS distal U/E test versus pinch grip in the MMT).

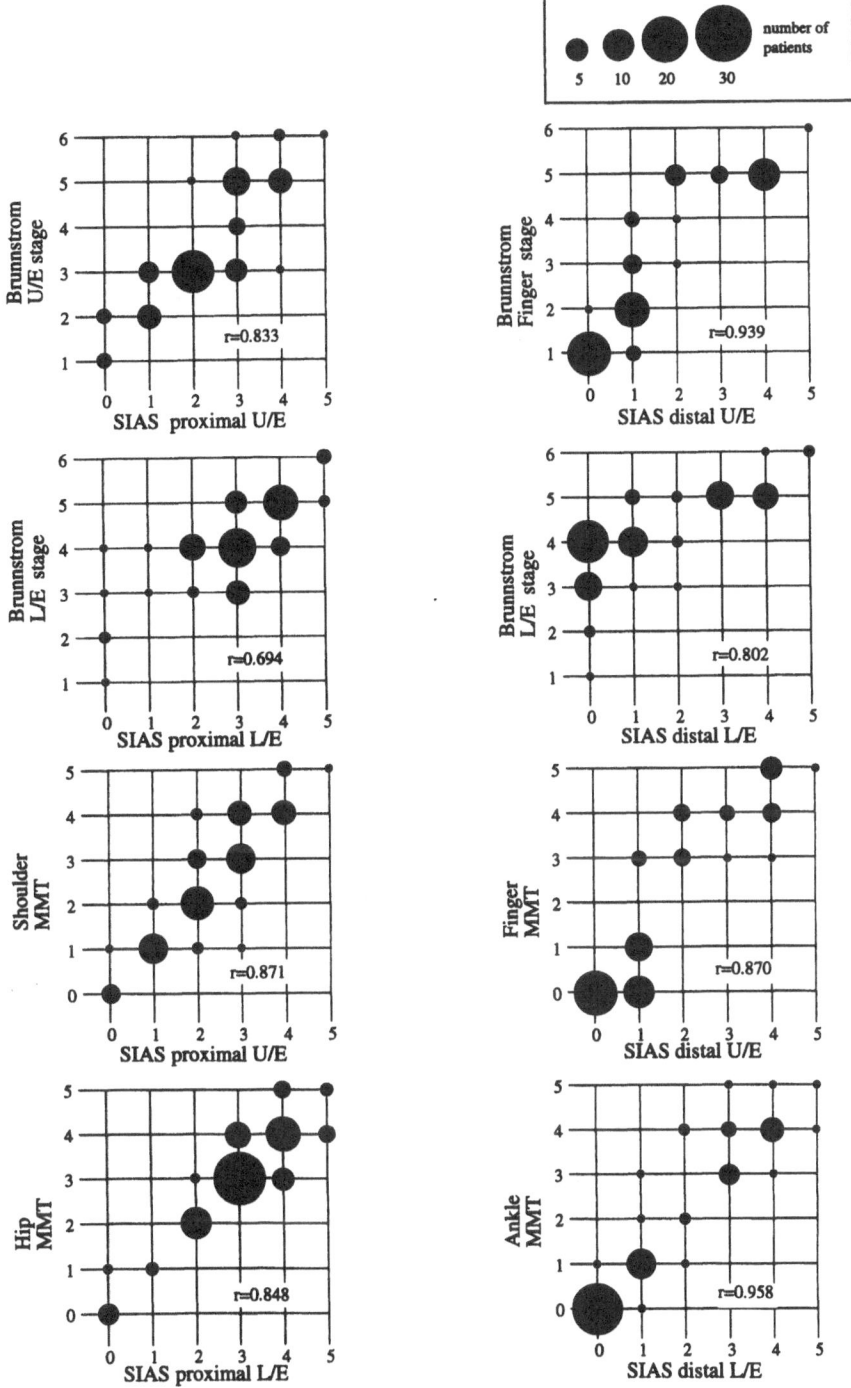

Fig. 1. Relationship between Stroke Impairment Assessment Set (SIAS) affected-side motor items and other motor assessment scales (*n* = 77). MMT, manual muscle testing; U/E, upper extremity; L/E, lower extremity; SIAS, stroke impairment assessment set; MMT, manual muscle set

In addition, our longitudinal study [12] indicated that many patients who remained in the same Brunnstrom stage or MMT level showed improvement in the SIAS-M. Therefore, the SIAS-M appeared to be more sensitive than the Brunnstrom stage or MMT for detecting the recovery of motor function in stroke patients.

Characteristics of the SIAS-M

To further investigate the SIAS-M, we examined the relationship between motor impairment and disability. The subjects, 65 stroke patients (mean age, 62.5 years), included 37 with cerebral hemorrhage and 28 with cerebral infarction (right brain damage, 37; left brain damage, 28). The time from onset ranged from 86 days to 270 months (median, 1090 days). Walking ability was assessed by the Functional Independence Measure (FIM) [13] score.

Table 2 shows the relationship between L/E function and walking ability using different scales. Proximal L/E (hip) function and distal L/E function were highly correlated with walking ability. However, the correlation of the Brunnstrom stage was lower than that of the MMT or SIAS, probably because the Brunnstrom L/E stage is a single scale that does not assess the proximal and distal extremity separately. Another reason may be that the Brunnstrom stage only assesses the pattern of movement, although muscle strength recovers when the ability to ambulate improves.

Figure 2 demonstrates the relationship between the SIAS distal U/E (finger) test and the U/E function score. The subjects were 99 stroke patients, including 45 with cerebral hemorrhage, 46 with cerebral infarction, and 8 with subarachnoid hemorrhage; mean age was 58.6 years; right brain damage had occurred in 50, left brain damage in 49. The duration from onset ranged from 164 days to 232 months (median, 182 days). The U/E function score consists of four activities of daily living (ADL) items for the affected-side upper extremity, including turning a page of a book, holding a bag, drinking with a glass, and pressing a sheet of paper on a desk. The score for each item is rated according to the degree of achievement of the task, with the lowest score being 0 and the full score being 10 points.

The distal U/E SIAS was strongly correlated with the U/E function score ($r = .905$). Grip strength was also strongly correlated with the U/E function score ($r = .763$).

Table 2. Spearman's rank correlation coefficients between motor impairment measured using different scales and walking ability ($n = 65$).

SIAS	
Proximal L/E (hip)	0.631
(knee)	0.594
Distal L/E	0.633
MMT	
Hip flexion	0.645
Knee extension	0.568
Ankle dorsiflexion	0.630
Brunnstrom stage	
L/E	0.575

L/E, lower extremity.

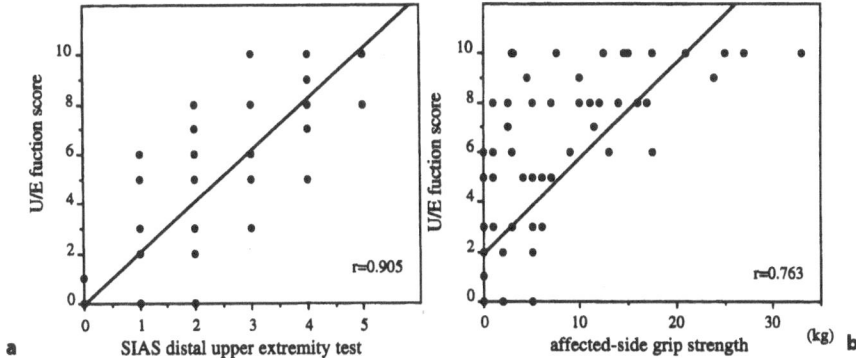

Fig. 2a,b. Relationship between motor impairment and upper extremity function (n = 99). a Relationship between SIAS finger test and upper extremity function score. b Relationship between grip power and upper extremity function score

However, a considerable number of the subjects with a low grip strength showed a high level of performance because they had good control of their fingers despite muscle weakness. For assessing such patients, a method that includes the concept of coordination is better than one based solely on muscle strength.

The MMT is a useful measure for stroke hemiplegia, and Sunderland et al. have reported that the grip strength should form a part of any adequate assessment battery [14]. However, our results indicate that SIAS is a better measure of finger function than grip strength.

Longitudinal Study of Motor Recovery Using the SIAS

Recovery of Affected-Side Function

To study the sensitivity of existing motor assessment scales in detecting the improvement of motor function in hemiplegics, we examined 24 stroke patients (12 with cerebral hemorrhage and 12 with cerebral infarction; mean age, 59.7 years; right brain damage, 15; left brain damage, 9) at 2–4 weeks, 4–8 weeks, and 8–12 weeks after onset using the SIAS-M, MMT, and Brunnstrom stage [12]. Among 24 patients, 17 showed improvement in ambulation when assessed with the FIM score. Among 17 patients, 11 (64.7%) showed no change in Brunnstrom stage, while only 5 (29.4%) showed no change in the SIAS motor score and 7 (41.2%) showed a constant MMT (Fig. 3). Knee and ankle function also changed in the SIAS and MMT, whereas the Brunnstrom stage has no individual items to evaluate knee or ankle function.

These results indicated that motor function actually recovered with the improvement in walking ability, and that the SIAS-M was sensitive enough to detect the change while the Brunnstrom stage was not. Therefore, we concluded that the Brunnstrom stage was less sensitive than the SIAS-M or MMT in detecting motor recovery after hemiplegia because it does not assess proximal and distal function separately.

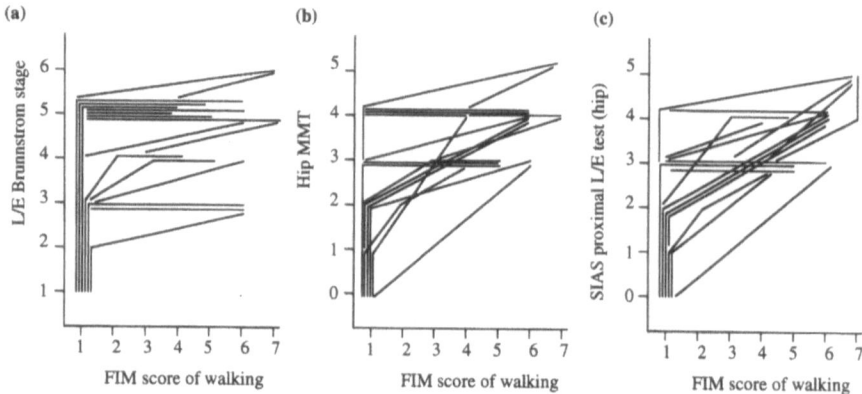

Fig. 3a–c. Relationship between lower extremity motor recovery and change in walking ability ($n =$ 17). The lower extremity motor function of the same subjects was assessed using the L/E Brunnstrom stage (a), the hip MMT (b), and the SIAS proximal L/E test (hip) (c). Note that more than half the patients showed a plateau in Brunnstrom stage while their walking ability was actually improving. FIM, functional independence measure.

Table 3. Longitudinal study of motor recovery using the SIAS-M[a].

		Scores on admission					
		0 (%)	(n)	1 (%)	(n)	2 (%)	(n)
Proximal U/E	Improved	10.5	(19)	68.8	(16)	100.0	(2)
	No change	57.9		6.3		0.0	
Distal U/E	Improved	3.7	(27)	54.6	(11)	100.0	(4)
	No change	59.3		45.5		0.0	
Proximal L/E (hip)	Improved	15.4	(13)	50.0	(6)	100.0	(11)
	No change	53.8		16.7		0.0	
Proximal L/E (knee)	Improved	20.0	(15)	40.0	(5)	100.0	(9)
	No change	13.3		20.0		0.0	
Distal L/E	Improved	4.2	(24)	33.3	(3)	100.0	(6)
	No change	75.0		33.3		0.0	

[a] The percentage of patients who showed improvement of 3 or more points at discharge and who showed no change for each SIAS-M item.
U/E, upper extremity; L/E, lower extremity.

Our study indicated that the SIAS-M is a reliable and sensitive method of assessing motor recovery after stroke. To observe motor recovery in stroke patients, we performed an additional longitudinal study using the SIAS-M. The subjects were 75 stroke patients (mean age, 63.3 years) studied within 6 weeks of admission to the rehabilitation hospital (29 had cerebral hemorrhage and 46 had cerebral infarction; right brain damage, 28; left brain damage, 47; duration from onset varied from 1 day to 44 months [median, 12 days]). The median length of stay was 45 days. Although the observation period varied, all the subjects stayed in hospital until their rehabilitation program was completed or motor recovery was finished.

Table 3 shows the percentage of patients who showed improvement of 3 or more points at discharge and who showed no change in each SIAS-M item. Only 3.7%–20%

of patients who were rated level 0 at admission improved to a level of 3–5 by discharge. Except for knee function, 53.8%–75.0% of the patients who were rated level 0 at admission did not improve at all. In contrast, 33.3%–68.8% of the patients who were rated level 1 at admission improved to a level of 3–5 by discharge. Only 6.3%–33.3% of the patients who were rated level 1 at admission (except for finger function) showed no change. There was a marked difference in recovery between level 0 (no voluntary movement) and level 1 (minimal movement) at admission for most of the SIAS-M items.

Compared with proximal function, distal function did not improve. In particular, 75% of the patients rated 0 for distal L/E function showed no change during rehabilitation. Therefore, we concluded that distal function improves less than proximal function as shown by Twitchell [15].

Among 11 patients with a rating of 1 on admission for distal U/E function, 8 subjects were rated 1A, which means mass flexion, and 3 subjects were rated 1C, which means minimal individual movement. A level of 1B, which means mass extension, was not observed on admission. Patients with a level of 1A at admission reached various levels by discharge. However, those with a level of 1C at admission always improved to a level of 3–5 by discharge. Although the numbers were rather small, we could at least conclude that finger function of level 1C at admission is an indicator of better recovery than level 1A function.

Change in Unaffected-Side Function

The SIAS assesses various aspects of stroke impairment. In addition to the SIAS-M, we consider that unaffected-side function is an important item. To validate the assessment of unaffected-side function, that is, to confirm whether unaffected-side impairment is present in stroke patients, we performed a longitudinal study using the same subjects as for the longitudinal study of the SIAS-M.

Table 4 shows the changes in unaffected-side function. Twelve of 75 patients improved their quadriceps score ($P < .01$, Wilcoxon signed rank test). In addition, unaffected-side grip strength showed an improvement at discharge of about 2 kg compared with that on admission ($P < .01$, paired t test). These results indicate that not only affected-side function but also unaffected-side function improves during the stay at a rehabilitation hospital.

Whether unaffected side function is impaired on admission or is strengthened at discharge is not clear, but we speculate that the unaffected side may also be impaired in the early stage of stroke because of the loss of ipsilateral innervation from the injured part of the brain [16].

Table 4. Changes in unaffected-side function ($n = 75$).

Unaffected-side quadriceps score		
+Ranks	12	$P < .01*$
−Ranks	0	
Unaffected-side grip power (kg)		
Admission	Mean, 23.51	SD, 11.84 ⎤ $P < .01**$
Discharge	Mean, 25.54	SD, 10.24 ⎦

* Wilcoxon signed-rank test.
** Paired t test.

In another study using stepwise regression analysis to investigate the concurrent relationship between impairment and disability [1], unaffected-side function was shown to be a necessary factor to explain the disability from impairment. Therefore, we concluded that unaffected-side function should be part of the SIAS. In other words, the "unaffected-side" function is actually also affected in stroke.

Discussion

Methods of assessing affected-side motor function can be classified into two groups: scales based on the synergy of movement and scales such as the MMT. Evaluation of affected-side motor function by assessing synergic movement cannot adequately describe the self-evident improvement of muscle strength and may also overlook the improvement of coordination. However, although the MMT reflects the number of recruited motor units, the recovery of coordination is not assessed. Furthermore, it is sometimes difficult to evaluate synergic movements such as elbow or finger flexion in combination with shoulder abduction. If one joint is fixed, other joints may also be affected. We consider that coordination and muscle strength should be included in a motor assessment scale without preventing assessment of the synergy of movement. The SIAS-M achieves this by employing both the concepts of synergy and the MMT.

The Motricity Index, the Canadian Neurological Scale (CNS) [17], and the National Institute of Health (NIH) stroke scale [18] are based on the concept of muscle strength (Table 5), and the patient is evaluated by observing the degree of achievement of a

Table 5. Comparison of various motor assessment scales for stroke patients[a].

	Number of tests[b]	Underlying concept	Other items
Global scale			
Canadian Neurological Scale	4	MMT	Level of consciousness, orientation, speech, facial palsy
National Institute of Healeth (NIH) scale	2	MMT	Level of consciousness, pupillary response, gaze, visual, facial palsy, plantar reflex, ataxia, sensory, neglect, dysarthria, language
Chedoke–McMaster Stroke Assessment	4	Synergy	Pain, postural control
Fugl-Meyer Score	50	Synergy	Sensation, ROM, pain
Stroke Impairment Assessment Set (SIAS)	5	MMT and synergy	Tone, DTR, sensory, pain, ROM, trunk, sound side, speech, visuospatial deficit
Motor assessment only			
Brunnstrom stage	>20	Synergy	None
Motricity Index	6	MMT	None

ROM, range of motion; DTR, deep tendon reflex.
[a] Assessment scales including disability were excluded.
[b] Number of tests for motor impairment of the affected-side limbs.

certain task against gravity or resistance. On the other hand, the Brunnstrom stage, Fugl-Meyer scale [19], and Chedoke–McMaster assessment [20] are based on the concept of synergy, so the patient is assessed by observing whether a task is accomplished with or without synergy.

Our cross-sectional and longitudinal studies demonstrated that the SIAS-M is sensitive enough to detect motor recovery in stroke patients. For upper extremity assessment, the SIAS-M is considered to be more useful than muscle strength scales, because muscle strength does not necessarily correlate with ADL in weak patients.

It is a problem that the Brunnstrom stage does not separate proximal and distal L/E function, although it separately assesses the proximal and distal upper extremity. As a result, important proximal L/E recovery may be missed after the achievement of ankle dorsiflexion task, making the Brunnstrom stage less sensitive for detecting motor recovery. Our conclusion is that although the Brunnstrom stage may be useful to describe gross phenomena in stroke patients in the therapeutic setting, its utility as a scale for assessing motor recovery or the efficacy of treatment is quite limited.

Another important problem is that the Brunnstrom stage and Motricity Index only assess motor impairment. In stroke research, such motor assessment scales have often been used as an indicator of the severity of stroke. However, stroke causes various types of impairment, and patients who have the same degree of motor impairment sometimes have quite a different level of disability according to the severity of their other impairments. Therefore, stroke research should be based on data obtained using a global stroke scale.

In addition, a global scale for stroke impairment is necessary to predict functional outcome. Our findings suggest that data on impairment is necessary to predict the future level of disability (see the chapter by Sonoda et al., this volume). The SIAS may be the minimum data set necessary for this purpose. The NIH scale, CNS, and Chedoke-McMaster scale are other global scales used for stroke outcome research, but they were not devised for use in the rehabilitation setting. For example, the CNS motor assessment items are scored by whether a certain muscle weakness is absent, mild, significant, or total. In the NIH scale, motor impairment is assessed by a task in which the patient holds the weaker leg raised to 30° for 5 s. Our longitudinal study of stroke patients showed that the CNS and the NIH scale were not sensitive enough to detect changes of motor impairment during rehabilitation (Seki M, Hase K, Domen K, Saitoh E, Chino N, unpublished data, 1994).

Another unique characteristic of the SIAS is that unaffected-side function is included. We have shown that the so-called unaffected side is actually also affected after a stroke. Even if not affected by the stroke itself, unaffected-side muscle strength may be reduced by aging and disuse. Because unaffected-side muscle weakness from any cause may impair functional independence, it should be measured as an important factor in the assessment of stroke impairment.

References

1. Domen K (1995) Reliability and validity of stroke impairment assessment set (the SIAS) (1): the items of affected-side motor function, muscle tone, deep tendon reflexes, and unaffected-side function (in Japanese with English abstract). Jpn J Rehabil Med 32:113–122
2. Wade DT (1992) Measures of motor impairment. Measurement in neurological rehabilitation. Oxford University Press, Oxford, pp 147–165

3. Wade DT (1992) Stroke scales. Measurement in neurological rehabilitation. Oxford University Press, Oxford, pp 291–306
4. Chino N, Sonoda S, Domen K, Saitoh E, Kimura A (1996) Stroke impairment assessment set (SIAS). In: Chino N, Melvin JL (eds) Functional evaluation of stroke patients. Springer, Tokyo, pp 19–31
5. Symposium recommendations for methodology in stroke outcome research. Stroke 21(suppl II):II-68–II-73
6. Sonoda S (1995) Reliability and validity of stroke impairment assessment set (SIAS) (2): the items comprise the trunk, higher cortical function, and sensory function, and effectiveness as outcome predictor (in Japanese with English abstract). Jpn J Rehabil Med 32:123–132
7. Domen K, Saitoh E, Sonoda S, Chino N, Kimura A, Liu M, Noda Y, Otsuka T (1993) Stroke impairment assessment set (SIAS) (2): reliability and validity of motor function assessment items of SIAS (in Japanese with English abstract). Jpn J Rehabil Med 30:310–314
8. Daniels L, Worthingham C (1986) Muscle testing techniques of manual examination, 5th edn. Philadelphia, Saunders
9. Domen K, Chino N, Sonoda S, Saitoh E, Kimura A (1991) Stroke impairment assessment set (SIAS). A preliminary report. Arch Phys Med Rehabil 72:770
10. Brunnstrom S (1970) Movement therapy in hemiplegia. Harper and Row, New York
11. Demeurisse G, Demol O, Robaye E (1980) Motor evaluation in vascular hemiplegia. Eur Neurol 19:382–389
12. Domen K, Saitoh E, Sonoda S, Chino N, Kimura A, Liu M, Noda Y, Otsuka T (1993) Stroke impairment assessment set (SIAS) (3): observation of motor recovery (in Japanese with English abstract). Jpn J Rehabil Med 30:315–318
13. Guide for use of the uniform data set for medical rehabilitation. Version 3.0. (1990) Data Management Service of the Uniform Data System for Medical Rehabilitation and Center for Functional Assessment Research, State University of New York at Buffalo, Buffalo
14. Sunderland A, Tinson D, Bradley L, Hewer RL (1989) Arm function after stroke. An evaluation of grip strength as a measure of recovery and a prognostic indicator. J Neurol Neurosurg Psychiatry 52:1267–1272
15. Twitchell TE (1951) The restoration of motor function following hemiplegia in man. Brain 74:443–480
16. Jones RD, Donaldson IM, Parkin PJ (1989) Impairment and recovery of ipsilateral sensory-motor function following unilateral cerebral infarction. Brain 112:113–132
17. Côté R, Battista RN, Wolfson C, Baucher J, et al (1989) The Canadian neurological scale. Neurology 39:638–643
18. Brott T, Adams HP, Olinger CP, Marler JR, et al (1989) Measurements of acute cerebral infarction: a clinical examination scale. Stroke 20:864–870
19. Fugl-Meyer AR, Jääskö L, Leyman I, Olsson S, et al (1975) The post-stroke hemiplegic patient. A method for evaluation of physical performance. Scand J Rehabil Med 7:13–31
20. Gowland C, Stratford P, Ward M, Moreland J, Torresin W, Van Hullenaar S, Sanford J, Barreca S, Vanspall B, Plews N (1993) Measuring physical impairment and disability with the Chedoke-McMaster stroke assessment. Stroke 24:58–63

Evaluation of Impairment and Disability in Stroke Patients: Current Status in Europe

Karl-Heinz Mauritz, Stefan Hesse, and Petra E. Denzler[1]

Summary. Evaluation of impairment and disability in stroke patients was introduced only recently in most European rehabilitation hospitals. However, there are initiatives in most countries to guarantee certain therapeutic quality standards. Unfortunately, there are large differences in the organization of stroke rehabilitation. Therefore, a unified database for impairment and disability evaluation does not exist on a European level. In this chapter, the most common evaluation instruments used in European countries are summarized. In addition, several examples are given for motor and cognitive impairments as well as for disabilities.

General Overview

Because there are many different health care systems in Europe, functional assessment of impairment and disability in stroke patients is quite divergent. Cultural differences are also large between southern and northern and between eastern and western countries, between Portugal and Sweden, or between France and Poland. There are countries with only state-owned hospitals (as in Sweden), and there are countries where almost all rehabilitation hospitals are privately owned (for example, Germany). Length of stay, the time of admission after the acute event, and the selection of patients also vary among countries and individual hospitals.

Overall it is probably fair to make the statement that, with the exception of Britain, the Scandinavian countries, and probably the Netherlands, assessment was introduced rather late in rehabilitation hospitals in Europe and in many places there is no quantification whatsoever. Among the leading groups in Europe to introduce assessment scales are the British groups in Oxford and in Bristol. Wade [1] published, fairly recently, a very important monograph about this subject that seems to have become the standard reference in Europe.

The lack of quantification in most European countries can be attributed to the fact that this was not required by paying agencies. Because rehabilitation in central European countries goes back to spas and recreational institutions, the only important item was client satisfaction. A similar situation certainly holds true for other Euro-

---

[1] Klinik Berlin, Department of Neurological Rehabilitation, Free University Berlin, Kladower Damm 223, Berlin 14089, Germany

Table 1. Required quality control criteria for rehabilitation facilities in Germany.

Structural quality
  Building
  Equipment (diagnostic and therapeutic)
  Staff and their qualifications
  Patient selection (diagnoses according to ICD)
Process quality
  Type, number, timing, and duration of therapies
  Single/group therapies
  Treatment goal and result
  Length of stay (LOS) (screening in a 3% sample)
Quality circles
  Within rehabilitation hospital
  External quality circles (documentation: time, frequency, participants, type of
    problem-solving strategy, etc.)
Patient satisfaction
  Sample of 15% are asked for their satisfaction 3 months after rehabilitation
Outcome quality
  Planned; not yet decided which scores

ICD, International Classification of Diseases.

pean countries. Therefore in most places the functional status of patients and patient outcome is only described and circumscribed in the discharge report.

However, the situation is now changing rapidly in most European countries. Paying agencies are starting to determine the quality and effectiveness of rehabilitation services. Health reforms to reduce health costs are planned or under way in several European countries. In Germany, for example, the federal pension insurance, which pays for a considerable percentage of rehabilitation costs, is introducing quality assurance procedures comprising structural quality (building, equipment, etc.) and process quality (number of therapies, etc.). There is no agreement yet about the necessary outcome quality measures and therefore outcome scales are not yet required. Table 1 summarizes the mandatory quality control criteria in German rehabilitation hospitals.

Surveying agencies unfortunately are usually not familiar with the excellent research work that has been done on assessment in such countries as the United States, Canada, United Kingdom, Sweden, Australia, and Japan. Therefore, many of the auditing and surveying agencies in Europe try to "reinvent the wheel" of assessment instead of utilizing the extensive experience gathered elsewhere (for a review, see [1]). Also, there is no unified database for rehabilitation at a European level, nor is there a database at a national level in most European countries. Therefore, it is difficult to present the state of the art of assessment in Europe. When screening publications of European origin, several differences between the U.S. data and most European countries are obvious: the case mix is quite different, and time of onset (the number of days from acute stroke until admission to a rehabilitation facility) is usually considerably longer in Western European countries. The later admission in most cases can be attributed to an oversupply of acute care hospital beds.

Length of stay also differs between countries. In Germany, Austria, and Switzerland the mean length of stay (LOS) is usually between 30 and 60 days. Figure 1 shows LOS data for stroke patients in the Berlin rehabilitation hospital, which seem to be repre-

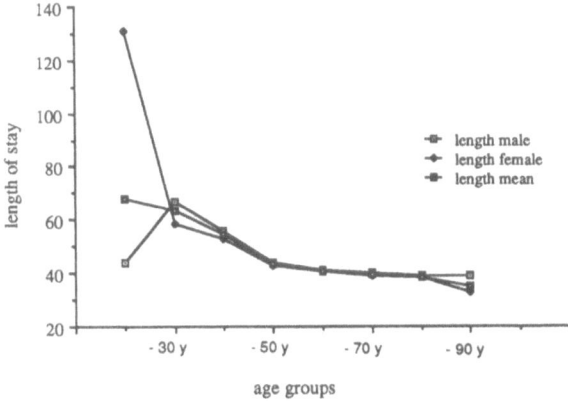

Fig. 1. Length of stay of stroke patients in a German neurologic rehabilitation hospital (Klinik Berlin, 1993) according to age groups. Average length of stay was 42 days

sentative for comparable units. Because they come later to rehabilitation, patients also score considerably higher at admission in their activities of daily living (ADL) levels in central European countries, compared to the United States or Great Britain. It seems that Japanese patients range in between.

Because there is a difference in payment according to the severity of the deficits, patients are often grouped into categories. In Germany, a phase model of rehabilitation was described by the association of pension funds. In that model (Fig. 2), patients are distributed into stages A through F. These stages are described only vaguely (Table 2), and no quantitative criteria are used. Similar models are used in other European countries.

Activitics of Daily Living Scales

Barthel Index

The most widely used ADL scale in Europe still is the Barthel index [2]. In Europe, the Barthel index has been tested extensively by British research groups [3,4]. Assessment is usually done by nurses or, in some places, also by occupational therapists. The improvement during an inpatient rehabilitation treatment shown in Fig. 3 for 120 patients of the Klinik Berlin corresponds very well with the results published by American rehabiliation hospitals [5]. Improvement in the single items of the Barthel index during a stroke rehabilitation also is comparable (Fig. 4).

Modified Barthel Indices

An Extended Barthel Index (EBI) was recently developed and is currently being tested in a multicenter-study in several European countries. According to Wade [6], "the main aim is to establish degree from any help, physical or verbal, however minor and for whatever reason." The index consists of 16 items, and each patient must be rated on all items. The rating on each item should be independent of ratings of other items. Physical transfer, for example, is a common element of item 5 (moving from wheel-

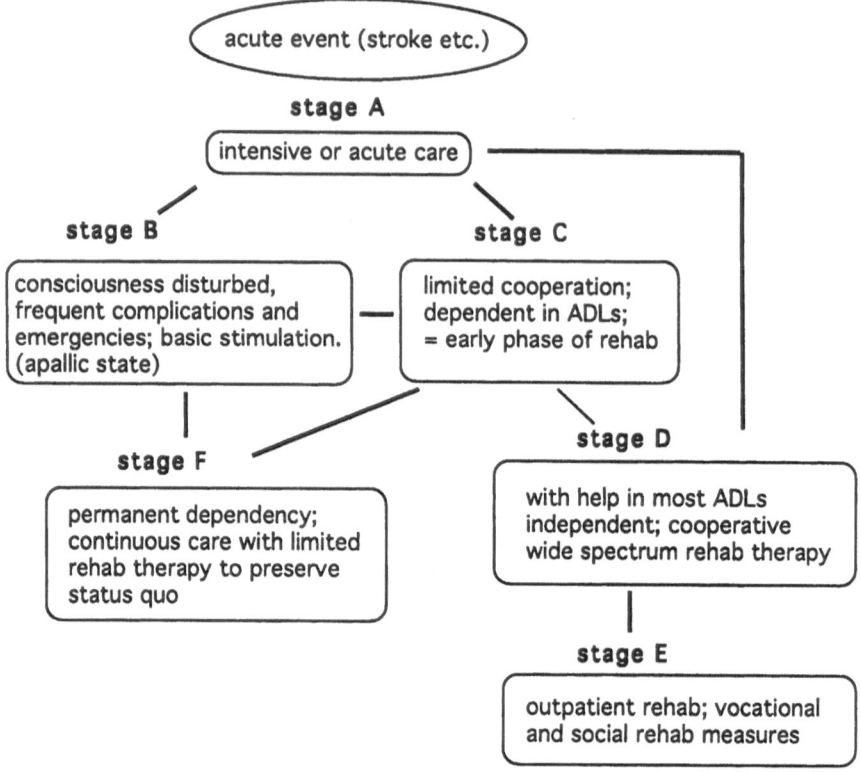

Fig. 2. Phase model of rehabilitation developed by German pension funds to separate patients into different stages (A–F). *ADL*, activities of daily living

Table 2. Stage model for neurological rehabilitation introduced by the association of German pension funds (VDR).

Stage A: Intensive and acute treatment (acute care unit)

Stage B: Disturbed consciousness; frequent complications and emergencies; basic stimulation (visual, acoustic, somatosensory, etc.); patients cannot cooperate; f.e. apallic syndrome; basic rehabilitation: swallowing, passive movements etc.; intensive care facilities should be on site

Stage C: Limited cooperation possible; however, dependent in activities of daily living (ADLs) (early stage of rehabilitation)

Stage D: Wide-spectrum rehabilitation treatment (with help in most ADLs independent)

Stage E: Outpatient rehabilitation; vocational and social reintegration

Stage F: Permanent dependency; continuous care with limited rehabilitation treatment (if patient could not proceed from stages B and C to more independence)

chair to bed), 8 (toilet), and 4 (bathing self). Items 11–16 are understanding of verbal or written instructions, questions and understanding of facial expressions and gestures (item 11), communicative abilities (item 12), social interaction (item 13), problem solving (item 14), learning, memory, and orientation (item 15), and visual

mean BI
100
90
80
70
60
50
40
30
20
10
0
47.5
58.6
69.1
77.7
Admission
Two weeks later
Four weeks later
At discharge

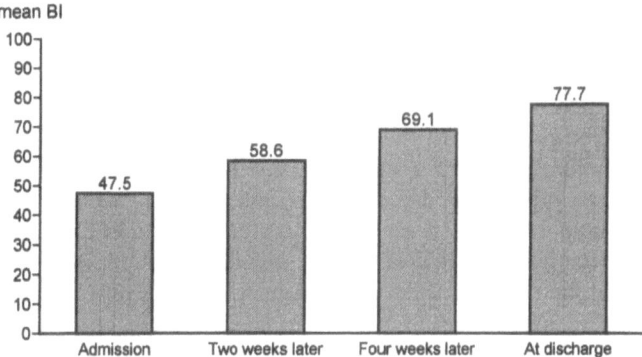

Fig. 3. Mean Barthel index (*BI*) at admission, 2 and 4 weeks later, and at discharge from an inpatient stroke rehabilitation program. Patients from Klinik Berlin, $n = 120$; mean BI difference, 30.6

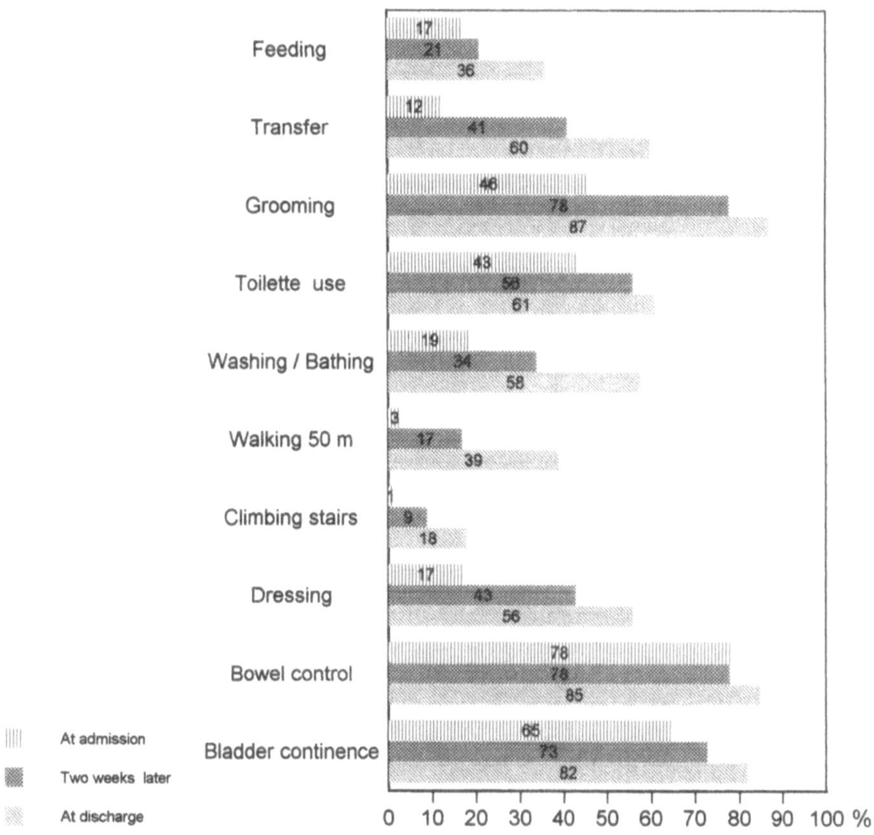

Feeding
17
21
36
Transfer
12
41
60
Grooming
46
78
87
Toilette use
43
56
61
Washing / Bathing
19
34
58
Walking 50 m
3
17
39
Climbing stairs
1
9
18
Dressing
17
43
56
Bowel control
78
78
85
Bladder continence
65
73
82
At admission
Two weeks later
At discharge
0 10 20 30 40 50 60 70 80 90 100 %

Fig. 4. Percentage of 120 patients independent at admission, 2 weeks later, and at discharge (average length of stay [LOS], 42 days) in the individual items of the Barthel index (BI)

perception/neglect. These additional items will be validated by an external expert rating (speech therapists, etc.).

It is planned to introduce a weighting of the individual items later (in manuscript) in which the EBI will be compared with the Functional Independence Measure (FIM) scale and the original Barthel Index. Each patient must be rated according to the degree of help that he actually requires. Furthermore, the index should be used as a record of what a patient does and not as a record of what a patient could do. Thus, it is of no importance whether this patient requires assistance because of physical, cognitive, or motivational deficits. A patient with severe motivational deficits may require major physical assistance or may require only supervision. His performance will therefore be rated either in the lowest or medium score, respectively. According to the *Manual for the Extended Barthel Index*, a patient may be considered as functionally independent only if he is able to perform the required task without assistance and within an appropriate time limit. Otherwise, he must be rated according to the degree of assistance that he requires to perform the task within sensible time constraints.

In England, assessment methods are more sophisticated than in any other European country, and the Barthel index was introduced earlier than in most other European countries [7]. Because of the limitations of the Barthel index, an Extended Activity of Daily Living Scale was created and validated as an overall assessment of functional independence in stroke patients discharged from hospital. Analysis of results of patients discharged from a stroke unit indicated that the four subsections (mobility, kitchen, domestic, and leisure) each formed a unidimensional hierarchical scale. Results also indicated that the scores from the subsections could be added to provide an overall score. The scale is suggested as appropriate for studies evaluating rehabilitation outcome after stroke and is suitable for postal surveys [8].

The Edinburgh prognostic score (incorporating measures of motor deficit, proprioception, and power) and the Orpington prognostic score (the Edinburgh score modified to include a measure of cognition) were developed to predict outcome in stroke rehabilitation. They were compared with the Barthel ADL scores at 1, 2, and 4 weeks after stroke and were correlated with outcome and patient Barthel ADL score at discharge. The authors concluded that the Orpington score when assessed 2 weeks poststroke is a useful prognostic indicator with special suitability for the elderly and may help to select patients most likely to benefit from stroke unit rehabilitation [9].

The Nottingham ADL index was designed originally for stroke patients. It is simple, reliable, hierarchically structured, and can be mailed as a questionnaire. It is also useful to monitor functional recovery [10].

Functional Independence Measure

Because the original Barthel Index does not take into account the cognitive aspects or communication deficits, other more comprehensive scale have been developed. One of the most successful assessment tools is the functional independence measure, FIM [11,12]: FIM includes self-care, sphincter control, mobility, locomotion, communication, and social cognition. FIM represents the burden of care. It is quantitative; 10 FIM points means 30–50 min of care. It is designed for inpatients and to be discipline free. Although several hundred hospitals are already using FIM in the United States, it is not yet widespread in Europe; the few institutions that are currently using FIM introduced it only 2 or 3 years ago.

In Sweden, there has been an increasing interest in FIM, and a translation into Swedish in 1991 was approved by the Uniform Data System in Buffalo. Initially, three Swedish rehabilitation departments contributed to FIM studies [13]: the rehabilitation hospitals in Danderyd, Huddinge, and Sahlgrenska. The University Department of Rehabilitation in Göteborg offers a 1-day introduction course, and a video presentation was also prepared. Because FIM is also of interest for a number of rehabilitation units in Sweden, it will probably be a uniform assessment scale in Sweden. There is close coooperation with the main rehabilitation hospital in Norway, Sunnaas Rehabilitation Hospital, and FIM has also been translated into Norwegian.

For the Swedish conditions, a Rasch analysis was performed [13] to make it comparable with a similar analysis performed in the United States. No significant difference was found between the difficulty of the individual items in Swedish and American rehabilitation hospitals. In Sweden, a comparative analysis of three different hospitals was also performed. Compared to the American data, patients in Sweden have higher functional levels at admission and discharge and on the average they are younger. Aside from this different case mix, there was good overall agreement in the data from the two countries. FIM assessment in Sweden is done only 1 week after admission to the hospital, whereas in the United States assessment is required within the first 72 h. In other European countries, the grading probably is also later done than in the United States.

In Italy, several groups now use FIM after Tesio in Milano began its use in 1993 with an Italian version [14]. Introductory courses are offered and examinations held; 157 persons were credentialed by April 1994 in Italy. As in many other European countries, admission to Italian rehabilitation hospitals is rather late because acute care hospitals are not pressed to discharge their patients. Therefore the average onset to admission time is 40 days, and as a consequence, the FIM admission score is higher than in the United States.

For France and Switzerland, a French version introduced in 1989 from Montreal is called MIF (mésure d'indépendence fonctionelle). Nurses are responsible for the assessment, as in most other countries.

In Germany, FIM was translated in 1992 by the team of the Klinik Bavaria, which also became a member of the Unified Data System (UDS). First results of assessments with FIM demonstrate that rehabilitation in this particular hospital starts rather late. Patients are admitted 16 months after the acute event and have an average FIM score of 108.7 on admission. The duration of inpatient treatment is 40 days, and the increase in FIM scores ranges from 4 to 14 points. In the Klinik Bavaria, 50% of the patients have admission scores of 120. A study done on these patients demonstrated that there is a high correlation between the Barthel index and the FIM. However, it also showed that in this functionally rather independent patient group the total FIM score is not very useful [15]. The FIM scale seems to be a valuable instrument for patients in postacute stages who are treated in Germany in specific rehabilitation hospitals like the Klinik Berlin.

Credentialing for the FIM is done at the Klinik Bavaria, and the German version is in first trial runs applied in a few rehabilitation hospitals in Austria and in German-speaking Switzerland (for example, in Lucerne). A comparison of FIM and the Extended Barthel Index has been started by hospitals in several countries.

In Portugal, the FIM was translated into Portugese and introduced in 1992 [16]. The admission score in Portugal is 72, and the discharge score is 101. In a follow-up 3 months later, patients score 108 points.

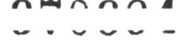

Katz Index of ADL

The predictive validity of the Katz index of Activities of Daily Living (ADL) regarding length of hospital stay, discharge to own home or death within 1 month, and its reproducibility in clinical practice was recently studied prospectively in Sodertalje and in Enkoping, Sweden [17]. The authors concluded that the instrument is now used as a valid tool for early prognosis of stroke outcome to facilitate the planning of care and rehabilitation in clinical practice. It seems, however, that the Katz index of ADL is used only rarely in Europe.

Kenny Index

The Kenny index of ADL was developed at the Sister Kenny Rehabilitation Institute in Minneapolis (Minnesota) in the 1960s [18]. It was one of the first quantitative assessment tools in rehabilitation and was still used in Israel at the Lowenstein Rehabilitation Centre, Raanana, until recently [19]. An assessment chart was developed that covered cognitive, basic, and integrated functions. When the results of the assessment using the chart were compared with those measured with the Kenny self-evaluation system, there was a positive correlation both between the Kenny system and the developed chart. It is of easy applicability, numerical scoring, and comprehensiveness; it is sufficiently sensitive to reflect the progress of patients during rehabilitation and enables reevaluation of initial treatment plans focusing on the needs of the individual patient.

Various Scales

There are many outcome studies on stroke rehabilitation in Germany or in Austria and Switzerland that apply questionnaires and scores not previously evaluated and validated [20]. For example, in a study done at the Neurological University Hospital in Vienna, the long-term prognosis of 310 patients suffering from ischemic stroke was investigated by means of questionnaires. It was the aim of the study to determine the predictive value of some clinical variables and symptoms in the subacute stage with respect to the familial and social functioning handicaps to be expected later. Between the number of strokes as well as the severity of some clinical signs (motor deficits, sensory deficits, speech disorders, organic mental syndrome) on the one hand, and the restrictions experienced in familial functioning on the other hand, a clear-cut correlation was found.

Similarly, in another German study a new score (IRES) was applied that was not validated by other groups [21]. The instrument enables essential parameters of rehabilitation patients' somatic, functional, and psychosocial status to be assessed and data collected at a "middle level of detail" in a standardized manner, that is, a patient questionnaire that can be used to complement medical assessment. Development and testing of the instrument has been supported during the past 3 years by a pension insurance fund, both financially and conceptually. The validation studies performed showed the instrument to be reliable, valid, and sensitive, and with good patient acceptance. Finally, a specifically designed computer program facilitates questionnaire data input and basic analyses. Some potential applications for the IRES questionnaire are seen in describing rehabilitation course and outcome, in documenting the effectiveness of rehabilitation measures (quality control), or in the framework of rehabilitation diagnosis.

In Switzerland, a functional scoring system was developed using a number of items in hierarchical order for gross function (13 items), leg and trunk (10 items), and arm (15 items). The test was applied at entry and at monthly intervals during treatment. The difference in scores before and after the rehabilitation program was statistically highly significant, irrespective of age and time interval between stroke and onset of treatment. Lower scores at entry necessitated longer rehabilitation [22].

Stroke Impairment Assessment Set

A new evaluation instrument for stroke patients, the Stroke Impairment Assessment Set (SIAS), has been described [23]. The individual items evaluate motor function, muscle tone, sensation, range of motion, pain, trunk control, visuospatial perception, aphasia, and functions on the unaffected side. Scores are plotted on a computer chart so that deficits can be identified immediately. There are plans to use the SIAS in several European rehabilitation units.

Measures of Motor Impairment

In 1987 the British Stroke Research Group recommended a set of measures for stroke patients. For motor impairment and disability, the following tests were chosen [1,6]:

Motor loss:	Motricity Index, Motor Club Assessment, Rivermead Motor Assessment
Mobility:	Functional Ambulation Categories (FAC)
Walking:	10-meter walk
Arm dexterity:	Nine- or Ten-hole Peg Test

These recommendations had little impact, however, on assessment in the clinical routine in many European rehabilitation hospitals outside Britain or Scandinavian countries, but assessment scales for motor impairment are used for scientific studies

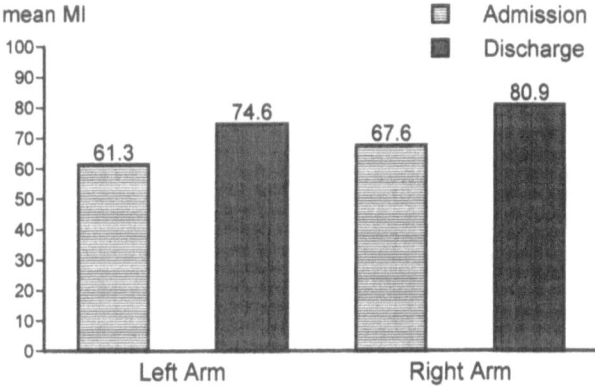

Fig. 5. Mean motricity index (*MI*) for right and left paretic arm at admission and discharge (average LOS, 42 days) in 120 patients. There is no difference between the two sides (mean ΔMI, 13.2)

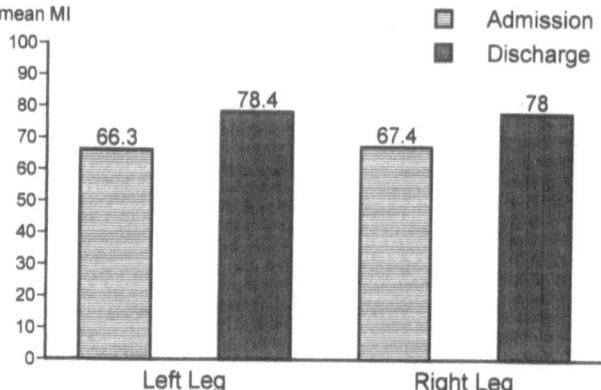

Fig. 6. Mean motricity index (*MI*) for right and left paretic leg at admission and discharge (average LOS, 42 days) in 120 patients. There is no difference between the two sides (mean ΔMI, 11.6)

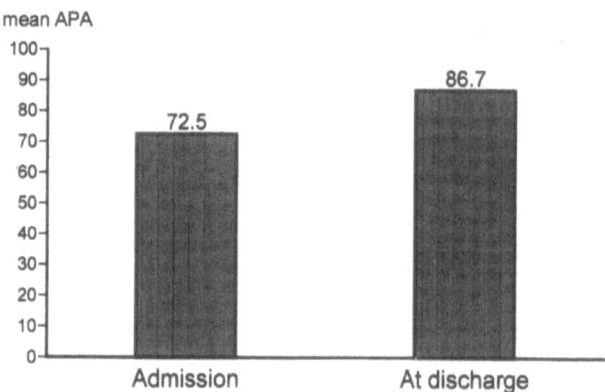

Fig. 7. Mean Ashburn physical assessment (*APA*) score for 100 patients at admission and discharge; mean APA difference, 14.2

measuring the effects of training procedures. Figures 5 and 6 demonstrate the improvement of the Motricity Index for the right and left arm and leg in 120 patients treated as inpatients for 6 weeks in the Klinik Berlin, and Fig. 7 shows the Ashburn Physical Assessment score for the same patient group.

In addition to dynamometry, the Motricity Index and the Trunk Control Test (TCT) are the assessment tools most often used for routine practice in stroke patients. Table 3 summarizes other assessment methods of motor impairment and disability collected from European literature. An asterisk indicates methods for which an apparatus is necessary.

The Fugl–Meyer Scale was shown recently to have its merits as a research tool with high overall reliability [24]. However, even for scientific studies the Rivermead Motor Assessment or the Motor Assessment Scale (MAS) are applied more often than the very detailed Fugl – Meyer assessment. In a newer development, Roque [25] proposed in Toulouse, France, the Toulouse Motor Scale for Stroke Patients that includes 41 items—trunk functions, autonomy in bed, leg functions, sitting, spasticity, arm

Table 3. Assessment of motor impairment/disability.

Force
  Medical Research Council (MRC) grades
  Dynamometry[a]
Tone
  Ashworth Scale for Spasticity
  Pendulum test
  Torque motors[a]
Posture
  Trunk Control Test (TCT)
  Force measuring platforms[a]
Gait
  Functional Ambulation Categories (FAC)
  Timed walking test
  Gait analysis[a]
    Ground reaction forces
    Joint angles
    EMG
Reaching/Grasping
  Action research arm test
  Nine-hole peg test (NHPT)
  Motorische Leistungsserie[a] (MLS)
Global Motor Scales
  Rivermead Motor Assessment (RMA)
  Motricity Index (MI)
  Fugl–Meyer Assessment Scale

[a] Use of apparatus required.

functions, and cooperation of patients among them. The scale was tested in several respects (kappa test reliability, test–retest and interrater reliability, internal correlation, correlation TCT or MAS, Frenchay arm test, finger-tapping test). According to the author, about 10–15 min are required to apply it. It has also been tested in Portugal [16]. However, it remains to be seen if there is a need for another motor scale.

Spasticity

Assessment of spasticity is especially difficult. For scientific studies, the Ashworth scale or recently more often the modified Ashworth scale [26] for grading spasticity is usually applied [27,28]. Other groups prefer the pendulum test.

Standing and Walking

Timed walking tests (10 m at ground level), walking endurance with self-adopted speed, and stair climbing (self-adopted speed with and without handrail, 90 steps each 16 cm high) are simple clinical measures that can also be used in more elaborate studies [29]. For gait rehabilitation the Functional Ambulation Categories (FAC) give details of the physical support needed by the patient. Because it is simple and has an established validity and reliability, it has been used in gait therapy studies by our group at the Klinik Berlin [30].

Table 4. Test batteries for cognitive and speech functions.

Cognitive functions
    Wechsler Adult Intelligence Scale (WAIS)
    Wechsler Memory Scale (WMS)
    Tübinger Luria-Christensen Test (TÜLUC)
    Rivermead Behavioral Inattention Test (RBIT)
    Rivermead Behavioral Memory Test (RBMT)
Speech functions
    Boston Aphasia Test (BAT)
    Porch Index of Communicative Ability (PICA)
    Aachener Aphasie Test (AAT)

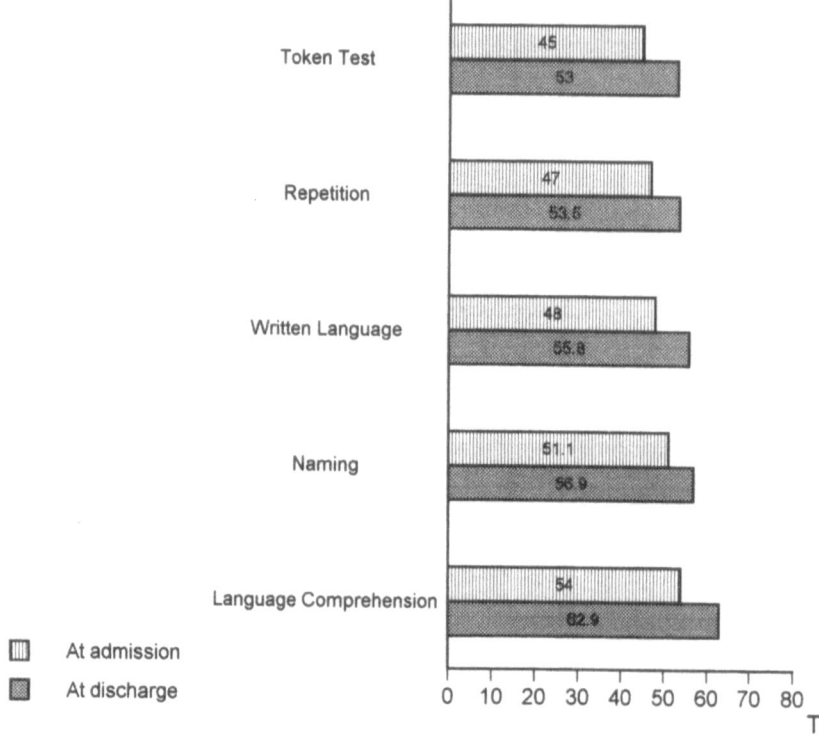

Fig. 8. Mean T values of the individual items of the Aachener aphasia test (AAT) at admission and discharge in 50 patients

Cognitive Assessment and Speech Functions

The British Stroke Research Group also recommended cognitive or neuro-psychological measures for stroke patients [1]:

Neglect: Albert's test and star cancelation
Level of consciousness: Glasgow coma scale
Visual field loss: Confrontation

Memory:	Rivermead Behavioral Memory Test, Wechsler Memory Scale
Perceptual problems:	Rivermead Perceptual Assessment Battery.
Aphasia:	Frenchay Aphasia Screening Test (FAST)
Orientation:	Orientation–Memory–Concentration Test

Several of these tests are used all over Europe. Some others that are commonly applied are compiled in Table 4. Major differences exist in the assessment of cognitive and communicative functions. For aphasia assessment, in German-speaking countries the most widely used aphasia test battery is the Aachener Aphasietest (AAT), which has been well standardized and which generates quantitative measures [31]. The AAT has also been adapted to the Dutch and Italian language A typical example of the AAT and its subitems in 50 aphasic patients is demonstrated in Fig. 8. For testing patients' communicative abilities in the acute phase, a bedside version (Aachener Aphasie Bedside Test, AABT) can be administered.

In the Netherlands, the Amsterdam-Nijmwegen-Everyday-Language-Test (ANELT) comprises ten items that test the patient for everyday communication situations [32]. Aphasia tests for several European languages were adapted from the Boston Diagnostic Aphasia Examination published by Goodglass and Kaplan [33]. In Norway, for example, Reinvang and Graves [34] published the Gruntest for Afasi.

Acknowledgments. We thank Dr. Schauer and Mr. Gahein-Sama for their help in collecting the data on stroke patients in the Klinik Berlin. Part of the work was supported by a research grant from the Gertrude-Reemtsma-Stiftung.

References

1. Wade DT (1992) Measurement in neurological rehabilitation. Oxford University Press, Oxford
2. Mahoney FL, Barthel DW (1965) Functional evaluation: the Barthel index. Md State Med J 14:61–65
3. Collin C, Wade DT, Davies S, Horne V (1988) The Barthel ADL index: a reliability study. Int Disabil Stud 10:61–63
4. Roy CW, Togneri J, Hay E, Pentland B (1988) An inter-rater reliability study of the Barthel index. Int J Rehabil Res 11:61–70
5. Granger CV, Hamilton BB, Gresham GE, Kramer AA (1989) The stroke rehabilitation outcome study. Part II: Relative merits of the total Barthel-Index score and a four-item subscore in predicting patient outcomes. Arch Phys Med Rehab 70:100–103
6. Wade DT (1992) Evaluating outcome in stroke rehabilitation (quality control and clinical audit). Scand J Rehabil Med (Suppl) 26:97–104
7. Kalra L, Smith DH, Crome P (1993) Stroke in patients aged over 75 years: outcome and predictors. Postgrad Med J 69:33–36
8. Lincoln NB, Gladman JR (1992) The extended activities of daily living scale: a further validation. Disabil Rehabil 14:41–43
9. Kalra L, Crome P (1993) The role of prognostic scores in targeting stroke rehabilitation in elderly patients. J Am Geriatr Soc 41:396–400
10. Barer DH (1989) Use of the Nottingham ADL scale in stroke: relationship between functional recovery and length of stay in hospital. J R Coll Physicians Lond 23:242–247
11. Granger CV, Hamilton BB, Sherwin FS (1986) Guide for use of the Uniform Data Set for Medical Rehabilitation. Uniform Data System for Medical Rehabilitation, Buffalo, New York

12. Granger CV, Hamilton BB (1994) The uniform data system for medical rehabilitation report of first admissions for 1992. Am J Phys Med Rehabil 73:51–55
13. Grimby G (1994) The functional independence measure (FIM) in Sweden. In: 7th World Congress of the International Rehabilitation Medicine Association, IRMA VII, Washington, DC
14. Tesio L (1994) Functional independence measure (FIM) in Italy. In: 7th World Congress of the International Rehabilitation Medicine Association, IRMA VII, Washington, DC
15. Frommelt P (1994) Functional independence measure in the Klinik Bavaria. In: 7th World Congress of the International Rehabilitation Medicine Association, IRMA VII, Washington, DC
16. Lains J, Caldas J, Azenha A, Oliveira R, Keating J (1994) Functional outcome in hemiplegics; a follow-up during one year. In: 7th World Congress of the International Rehabilitation Medicine Association, IRMA VII, Washington, DC (Abstract F 195)
17. Asberg KH, Nydevik I (1991) Early prognosis of stroke outcome by means of Katz index of activities of daily living. Scand J Rehabil Med 23:187–191
18. Schoening HA, Iversen IA (1968) Numerical scoring of self-care status: a study of the Kenny self-care evaluation. Arch Phys Med Rehabil 49:221–229
19. Feder M, Ring H, Rozenthul N, Eldar R (1991) Assessment chart for inpatient rehabilitation following stroke. Int J Rehabil Res 14:223–229
20. Oder W, Binder H, Baumgartner C, Zeiler K, Deecke L (1988) Zur Prognose der sozialen Reintegration nach Schlaganfall. Rehabilitation (Stuttg) 27:85–90
21. Gerdes N, Jackel WH (1992) "Indikatoren des Reha-Status (IRES)"—Ein Patientenfragebogen zur Beurteilung von Rehabilitations-bedürftigkeit und -erfolg. Rehabilitation (Stuttg) 31:73–79
22. Kesselring J, Gamper UN (1992) Vom Nutzen der Neurorehabilitation. Versuch einer Quantifizierung am Beispiel von 312 Schlaganfallpatienten in der Klinik Valens. Schweiz Med Wochenschr 122:1206–1211
23. Chino N, Sonoda S, Domen K, Saitoh E, Kimura A (1994) Stroke impairment assessment set (SIAS)—a new evaluation instrument for stroke patients. Jpn J Rehabil Med 31:119–125
24. Sanford J, Moreland J, Swanson LR, Stratford PW, Gowland C (1993) Reliability of the Fugl-Meyer assessment for testing motor performance in patients following stroke. Phys Ther 73:447–454
25. Roques C (1994) Motor function assessment for hemiplegic patients. In: 7th World Congress of the International Rehabilitation Medicine Association, IRMA VII, Washington, DC (abstract)
26. Bohannon RW, Smith MB (1987) Interrater reliability of a modified Ashworth scale of muscle spasticity. Phys Ther 67:206–207
27. Hummelsheim H, Mauritz KH (1993) Neurophysiological mechanisms of spasticity modification by physiotherapy. In: Thilmann A, et al (eds) Spasticity: mechanisms and management. Springer, Berlin Heidelberg, pp 426–438
28. Hesse S, Friedrich H, Domasch C, Mauritz KH (1992) Botulinum toxin therapy for upper limb flexor spasticity: preliminary results. J Rehabil Sci 5:98–101
29. Hesse S, Jahnke MT, Schreiner C, Mauritz KH (1993) Gait symmetry and functional walking performance in hemiparetic patients prior to and after a 4-week rehabilitation programme. Gait Posture 1:166–171
30. Hesse S, Bertelt CH, Schaffrin A, Malezic M, Mauritz KH (1994) Restoration of gait in nonambulatory hemiparetic patients by treadmill training with partial body-weight support. Arch Phys Med Rehabil 75:1087–1093
31. Huber WK, Poeck K, Weniger D, Willmes K (1983) Der Aachener Aphasie-Test. Hogrefe, Göttingen
32. Blomert L, Koster C, van Mier H, Kean ML (1987) Verbal comunication abilities of aphasic patients: the everyday language test. Aphasiology 1:463–474
33. Goodglass H, Kaplan E (1972) The assessment of aphasia and related disorders. Lea and Febiger, Philadelphia
34. Reinvang I, Graves R (1975) A basic aphasia examination: description with discussion of first results. Scand J Rehabil Med 7:129–135

Rehabilitation and Functional Evaluation of the Stroke Survivor in New Jersey

Thomas W. Findley[1,2], Richard D. Zorowitz[1,2], Miriam Maney[2], and Mark V. Johnston[1,2]

Summary. The care of stroke survivors presents significant challenges both in the state of New Jersey and in the United States. Over 500 000 new cases of stroke yearly join the nearly three million stroke survivors in the United States. Stroke rehabilitation must address the medical, functional, vocational, avocational, and psychological issues of the stroke survivor using an interdisciplinary team of skilled professionals. This chapter describes admission criteria for inpatient stroke rehabilitation and guidelines for the assessment and treatment of the stroke survivor in various areas such as mobility and locomotion, activities of daily living (ADLs), community management, speech–language and cognitive disorders, and common medical complications. A model for functional evaluation used in the stroke rehabilitation program is described. Finally, functional data from 1900 stroke survivors admitted to the stroke rehabilitation program between January 1, 1992, and June 30, 1994, are described. While onset-to-admission intervals and legnth of stay have declined over the period, the functional status of the stroke survivors at discharge has remained constant. The efficiency of functional gains attained during the rehabilitation stay, as well as the efficiency of cost relative to these functional gains increased during the study period. The trends illustrated by these data reflect a movement by third-party payers to cap patient care costs by imposing shorter rehabilitation stays and shifting care to less intensive settings such as subacute units, nursing home facilities, and home care. However, rehabilitation professionals still must address the continuing need to maximize function and the safety of stroke survivors while meeting the demands of the government and insurance industry.

Introduction

Stroke remains one of the most serious neurological problems in the United States today. It is the third most common cause of death, and stroke patients constitute more than half the patients hospitalized for neurological problems in community hospitals [1]. Approximately 500 000 new cases of stroke, of which 40% are fatal, occur each

[1]Department of Physical Medicine and Rehabilitation, University of Medicine and Dentistry (UMDNJ)-New Jersey Medical School, 150 Berger Street, Newark, NJ 07103, USA
[2]Kessler Institute for Rehabilitation, 1199 Pleasant Valley Way, West Orange, NJ 07052, USA

year. New stroke victims join the approximately 3 million stroke survivors alive in this country. Of patients who survive a stroke past 30 days, 50% are still alive after 7 years [2]. The cost of patient care and earnings lost from stroke totaled $30 billion in 1993 [3].

Likewise, stroke presents a significant challenge in New Jersey (United States). In 1992, the New Jersey State Department of Health reported that 61065 patients were discharged from acute care hospitals with a primary or secondary diagnosis of stroke, for an overall rate of 7.8 per 1000. Half of these, or 28500, had the primary diagnosis of stroke. During 1992, 880 patients from northern New Jersey were admitted to the Kessler Institute for Rehabilitation in West Orange, NJ, for intensive, comprehensive rehabilitation; Kessler Institute has the majority, 300 of 330, licensed inpatient rehabilitation beds in northern New Jersey. This chapter describes in detail our experience with stroke rehabilitation.

Stroke rehabilitation at Kessler involves an interdisciplinary, comprehensive approach that addresses medical, functional, and psychosocial issues. The team includes the patient and significant family members, a physiatrist, rehabilitation nurse, physical therapist, occupational therapist, speech-language pathologist, social worker, psychologist, and vocational counselor. From the day of admission, the team evaluates the patient and begins the process of improving functional skills. In the past, patients may have remained on the stroke rehabilitation unit until their functional abilities reached a plateau. However, as lengths of stays have declined in inpatient rehabilitation, the goal of the rehabilitation stay has shifted to one in which patients improve their functioning to the point that they can be safely discharged to their homes, in the care of their family and others, without undue stress. The ability of the family to provide patient care needs to match the functional level of the patient to prevent patient deterioration or excess burdens that affect the health and welfare of family members. Scales of family help available are currently being developed at our institution to assist with matching of the help required by the patient with the help the family can provide [4]. In the new system, whenever possible rehabilitation continues after discharge via outpatient clinics and home visits by nurses and therapists.

This chapter describes the means by which patients are selected for inpatient stroke rehabilitation and are assessed functionally by the interdisciplinary team to maximize a suitable discharge to their home. Although some persons who provide assistance in the home may be unrelated to the patient, all such persons are termed "family members" in this discussion. In addition, program evaluation data are presented that illustrate wider, nationwide trends in stroke rehabilitation.

Admission Criteria

Stroke rehabilitation admission criteria are designed to help identify those stroke survivors who might best benefit from a comprehensive inpatient rehabilitation program. At the same time, these criteria help reduce denials in reimbursement from third-party payers for inpatient services. Patients who are not candidates for inpatient rehabilitation are referred to other levels of care, such as visiting nurse services, outpatient services, nursing homes, or subacute rehabilitation facilities.

Candidates for inpatient stroke rehabilitation generally must demonstrate the likelihood that they will be discharged from the rehabilitation facility to their home.

Important predictors of good rehabilitation outcome for stroke survivors include stable medical condition; adequate family and social support; and demonstration of significant motor, cognitive, and functional skills early during the course of recovery from the stroke [5]. The patient must be able to tolerate a minimum of 3 h per day of therapy, including physical therapy and occupational therapy. Speech therapy and psychological or social services also may be provided. At the time of admission, the stroke survivor must require the assistance or supervision of a caregiver in at least two of the following areas: mobility; activities of daily living (ADL); bladder and/or bowel incontinence; cognitive, communication, or perceptual impairment; and medical complications, such as spasticity, contractures, pressure sores, bladder dysfunction, pain, or other conditions which require that the patient be educated in the proper management of the condition to avoid current or future complications. In addition, similar treatment must not have been completed previously in a comprehensive rehabilitation facility. A patient may not be readmitted to rehabilitation unless his or her circumstances have changed or the patient condition indicates potential for reaching previously unattained goals.

Past guidelines have stated that a stroke survivor must be able to demonstrate the potential for functional improvement to be admitted to an intensive inpatient stroke rehabilitation program. Prerequisites included responsiveness to verbal and visual stimuli, sufficient mental alertness to participate in the rehabilitation program, and a premorbid condition that indicates a potential for rehabilitation. However, these criteria are no longer sufficient if a stroke survivor has the family or social support systems allowing for a discharge to home where further functional improvement may occur. Our guidelines currently assess the patient–family unit for potential for improvement. In some cases, treatment objectives in rehabilitation focus more on equipment evaluation and on family training in patient care than on improving the functional skill of the patient per se. While the patient may return home requiring less assistance than before admission, this may not be the primary factor in determining timing of discharge.

Mobility and Locomotion

For most stroke survivors, probably the most important priority is ambulation. Prerequisites for training in ambulation include the ability to follow commands; adequate trunk control for sitting and standing; minimal or no contractures of the hip flexor, knee flexor, and ankle plantarflexor muscles; and muscle strength adequate to stabilize the hip and knee joints.

Physical therapy, occupational therapy, and nursing participate in the evaluation of mobility and locomotion. Gait training begins by teaching transfers to the bed, mat, and wheelchair. The patient must be able to bear weight consistently on the affected extremity. Standing balance must be maximized using visual, proprioceptive, or labyrinthine cues. The patient is taught the optimal pattern of gait on parallel bars, without bars, and on stairs, ramps, and curbs.

Stroke survivors may require orthoses to normalize their gait and to improve mobility and safety in ambulation. An orthotics clinic has been organized to evaluate the patient and issue the best possible orthotic device for that patient. The clinic comprises a physiatrist, physical therapist, and orthotist. A number of different orthotics may be evaluated on the patient before a decision for the definitive orthotic is made. The clinic allows for a number of patients to be evaluated at the same time and thus optimizes the time of the professionals involved to provide these services. Also, 40% of our stroke patients are provided leg braces, usually plastic molded ankle-foot orthoses.

Patients who have limited or no ability to ambulate require a wheelchair for mobility. A wheelchair clinic operates to evaluate the stroke survivor and to provide the most appropriate wheelchair for the patient. The wheelchair clinic is staffed by a physiatrist, occupational therapist, and a wheelchair vendor. Different types of wheelchairs may be loaned to the patient for trials. Lightweight wheelchairs or motorized wheelchairs may be issued to appropriate patients with approval from their third-party payers.

Once orthotics, assistive devices, and wheelchairs have been issued, the patients are allowed to use these inside and outside the rehabilitation hospital with permission of the attending physiatrist. The therapists train family members in the proper assistance or supervision of mobility activities and in use of the equipment. Nursing staff may assist or supervise the patients in ambulation on the nursing unit, and family members may assist or supervise the patient in ambulation outside the hospital during a therapeutic functional trial ("day pass").

Activities of Daily Living

Stroke survivors frequently do not place the same degree of importance on self-care ADLs as they place on ambulation. Teaching ADLs may be more difficult than teaching ambulation because the affected upper limb is less functional than the affected lower limb. Performance of ADLs requires visual, cognitive, perceptual, and coordination skills in addition to range of motion, motor strength, and sensation. As a result, the occupational therapist and speech-language pathologist typically collaborate in teaching compensatory strategies for performing ADLs in the face of these deficits.

One unique aspect of the evaluation and training of ADLs at Kessler is Independence Square, an indoor therapy environment that replicates real-life activities which patients encounter on return to the community. This environment is composed of several settings: an apartment, including kitchen, bedroom, and bathroom; a market; a bus, including stairs and a wheelchair lift; and a bank. An ambulation course incorporates many of the surface variations and levels that are encountered during community ambulation: grass, sidewalk, concrete, and curbs. Stroke survivors are able to practice tasks in strikingly realistic settings before attempting them in their actual environment. Patients also may evaluate their ability to perform ADLs in selected settings outside the rehabilitation hospital.

Group training provides opportunities for stroke survivors with cognitive, perceptual, or communicative impairments to develop cognitive, communicative, and functional skills. Communication–functional skills groups provide opportunities for stroke survivors to plan and execute activities such as a meal or a trip with other persons having similar deficits. Patients may apply learned skills in the community life skills group, which supervises functional trips to locations such as a food store, laundromat, post office, or restaurant. Nurses also encourage the patient to use newly learned skills on the nursing unit to reinforce patient independence. The therapists and nurses train family members in the proper assistance and supervision of all aspects of self-care activities, including medications administration. Family members then may assist or supervise the patient in these activities outside the rehabilitation hospital during a therapeutic functional trial.

Driving

Driving is an important goal for some stroke victims. New Jersey is one of only seven or eight of the United States that require physicians by law to notify the Division of Motor Vehicles that a patient has suffered a stroke. Once notified, the Division of Motor Vehicles requests that the physiatrist or other physician medically clear the patient for driving. The physician must determine whether the stroke survivor can or cannot operate an adapted or unmodified vehicle. If the physician determines that the patient has sufficient motor or cognitive deficits that require formal evaluation, the patient may be referred for evaluation. Kessler has had a driving evaluation and training program for 30 years. Occupational therapy at Kessler administers a predriving evaluation that tests basic cognitive skills needed for driving, such as memory, spatial organization, attention, concentration, and reaction times. Driving skills are tested in a simulator or behind the wheel with an instructor. Adaptive aids, such as steering wheel pegs and accelerator extensions, may be incorporated to compensate for motor deficits, and the patient may receive driving lessons to learn how to use the equipment. Once a patient has received clearance from the physician or has successfully completed the driving program, the patient must appear for and pass a standard driving test given by the Division of Motor Vehicles. Fifteen percent of our stroke patients undergo formal driving evaluation at Kessler.

Return to Work

Twenty-five percent of our stroke rehabilitation patients are under age 65, and approximately one-third of these are able to return to work. To return to work, patients must overcome motor, cognitive, perceptual, and communication deficits. Physical therapists may evaluate and teach the stroke survivor mobility skills necessary for employment. Occupational therapists and speech-language pathologists may train the patient in prevocational skills, such as ADLs and cognition, perception, and communication. Neuropsychologists may evaluate cognitive skills in great detail to determine the nature and degree of cognitive deficits that influence the feasibility of returning to work. If cognitive deficits are significant, the patient may be enrolled in a cognitive remediation program, subject to approval by third-party payers. The cognitive remediation program consists of an occupational therapist, a speech therapist, a recreational therapist, neuropsychologists, a vocational counselor, and rehabilitation aides. They work in a close-knit, interdisciplinary team to evaluate and train the patient in compensatory strategies for cognitive and practical problems. The program is customized to the needs of the patients. Both individual and group treatments are provided.

Vocational counselors obtain work histories from patients. However, their effectiveness in assisting the patient to return to work is limited as third-party reimbursement usually is not available. As a result, many stroke survivors are referred to the state Division of Vocational Rehabilitation (DVR). DVR works with the physiatrist in determining what services are required to improve prevocational as well as vocational skills. They will fund physical therapy, occupational therapy, and speech therapy for limited durations. They will also fund neuropsychological and driving evaluations. If needed, they will fund work capacity assessments, work hardening, and onsite evaluations in conjunction with the industrial rehabilitation department. DVR generally acts as a liaison between the physician, the patient, and the workplace, and helps to modify the work environment so that the patient may return to gainful employment.

Speech-Language and Cognitive Disorders

Speech and language disorders may be assessed by both formal testing and conversational interaction. Formal tests of language impairments (i.e., aphasia, apraxia, dysarthria, cognitive-communication impairment) may be made using commercially available testing batteries. As the two are entwined, cognitive dysfunction often is tested along with language dysfunction. Hemineglect is routinely assessed by occupational therapists, who observe how the patient uses his afflicted side in therapeutic exercises and self-care activities, as well as using items from formal tests. Patients may receive therapy individually or may be enrolled in group activities to enhance recovery and the learning of compensatory skills.

Common Medical Complications

Every stroke patient admitted to the rehabilitation unit must be considered for secondary prophylaxis of stroke. While aspirin currently is the standard medical therapy for secondary prophylaxis of nonhemorrhagic stroke, ticlopidine appears to be more effective than aspirin [6,7]. It is especially indicated for patients who have failed aspirin therapy or cannot take aspirin [8]. Dipyridamole has not been shown to be effective alone or with aspirin but may be indicated in patients with prosthetic heart valves or arterial bypass grafts [9,10]. Warfarin may be indicated in patients with prosthetic heart valves or atrial fibrillation. Studies of pentoxifylline are still inconclusive [11]. Secondary prophylaxis of hemorrhagic stroke includes control of etiological factors such as hypertension [12].

Deep venous thrombosis (DVT) may occur in 30%–60% of stroke survivors. Clinical signs and symptoms such as pain, swelling, and warmth of the extremity are at best marginally diagnostic. Clinical suspicion should be raised in the hemiplegic patient who is not ambulatory within 3 months of stroke onset. Noninvasive testing, such as Doppler and impedance plethysmography, is therefore a routine part of diagnosis. Prophylactic measures should be taken for patients at risk for DVT. Prophylaxis may be discontinued once the patient is ambulating consistently in or outside the parallel bars [13].

Strokes may disinhibit the reflex mechanisms for emptying the bowels. Sensory or cognitive impairments may prevent control of defecation. Diets should include adequate fluids and fiber, and adjunctive medications should be given as necessary. Patients should be toileted after meals to take advantage of the gastrocolic reflex. Stool softeners and bowel stimulants may be prescribed as necessary.

A variety of voiding disorders may be observed after stroke. Reversible causes, such as urinary tract infection, fecal impaction, and reduced mobility, should be evaluated and treated. Postvoid residual urine volumes should be measured to assess for urinary retention. Symptoms of urinary incontinence, frequency, and urgency should be noted. At Kessler, patients with voiding dysfunction are referred for urodynamic studies to characterize the voiding disorders and to determine appropriate intervention. One-quarter of our stroke patients undergo such urodynamic studies [14].

Swallowing dysfunction, or dysphagia, may occur in as many as one-third of patients with cortical or brainstem lesions [15]. Dysphagia should be suspected in patients with impaired cognition, nasal regurgitation, coughing, "gurgly" voice, or impaired cough associated with the absence of bilateral gag reflex [16,17]. Evaluation of dysphagia is delegated to nurses, dietitians, occupational therapists, and speech-language pathologists. Nurses evaluate every patient on admission to the nursing unit to determine whether any swallowing problem exists. If a swallowing problem is discovered, the team discusses the problem and decides which disciplines need to treat or further evaluate the patient. The occupational therapist may evaluate the patient if a problem with feeding, such as unilateral neglect or impulsivity, is discovered. The speech-language pathologist becomes involved with the patient if a suspicion of aspiration is raised. On their recommendation, a videofluorographic swallowing study (VFSS) of liquids, purees, and solids is undertaken to identify the swallowing disorders and organize a treatment plan. The dietary plan is organized and executed by the dietitian, who can incorporate admission laboratory data into the dietary recommendation. Nonoral feedings by gastrostomy or jejunostomy may be necessary if oral nutritional needs cannot be met. We currently perform VFSS studies on 16% of our patients with stroke.

The patient may self-feed or be fed in different settings, depending on the level of safety and need for supervision or assistance. Patients requiring individual attention may be fed on the nursing unit by a nursing aide, nurse, occupational therapist, or speech-language pathologist. Patients requiring supervision may be enrolled in the breakfast or lunch groups, which are supervised by occupational therapists. If a patient can feed independently, he is medically cleared to eat in the communal patient dining room.

Functional Evaluation

Throughout the inpatient rehabilitation stay, the function of the patient is monitored and formally evaluated by the team periodically to justify the necessity of inpatient rehabilitation stay. The team meets within 1 week after a patient is admitted and records the admission functional status of the patient. Evaluations are performed in a problem-oriented format to allow the input of all appropriate disciplines. The length of the rehabilitation stay is projected, and goals are set, bearing in mind family and patient desires. Key family members and the patient, when appropriate, are invited to attend the initial evaluation conference and to participate in the setting of goals, and are given the opportunity to ask questions of the team. The ideal is that family (and patient) participate as members of the rehabilitation team. Following this conference, the team holds a reevaluation conference every 1–2 weeks, depending on the needs of the patient. At each conference, functional gains are documented, and short-term and long-term goals are reviewed.

Functional progress is recorded using the functional independence measures (FIM). The FIM requires therapists to rate patient disability in 18 activities, including mobility, self-care ADLs, continence, communication, and cognition [18]. Each activity is rated according to a seven-level scale that ranges from total independence at the top (a score of 7) to total dependence/inability at the bottom (a score of 1).

The use of FIM data permits the evaluation of the stroke program in relation to national and regional norms. This program evaluation system demonstrates our

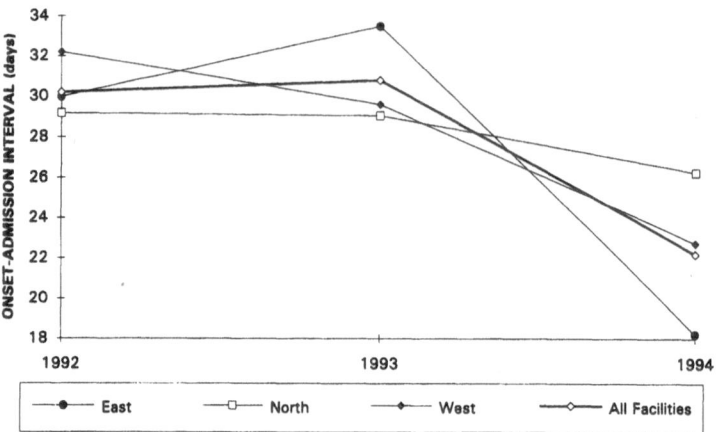

Fig. 1. Patient chronicity in terms of onset–admission interval (OAI) (number of days from onset to rehabilitation admission at three Kessler Institute facilities

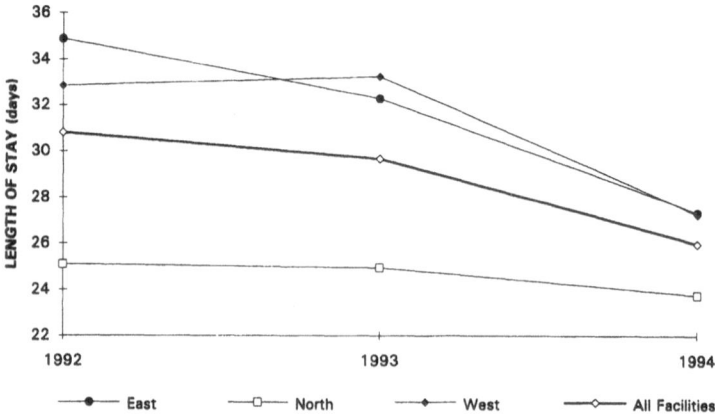

Fig. 2. Length of stay (LOS) in days at each facility

patient outcomes and affirms the quality and effectiveness of our services. Because Kessler consists of three separate facilities, the data also permit a quantitative comparison among the facilities. In the long run, this program evaluation system should help us to identify better techniques to improve functional status and optimal levels of function at discharge, balancing patient and family need against financial constraints.

A Statistical Description of Kessler

Retrospective data were collected from 1900 patients admitted to the three facilities of the Kessler Institute for Rehabilitation between January 1, 1992, and June 30, 1994: East (East Orange, NJ), North (Saddle Brook, NJ), and West (West Orange, NJ). Data that are routinely collected on each patient include the following:

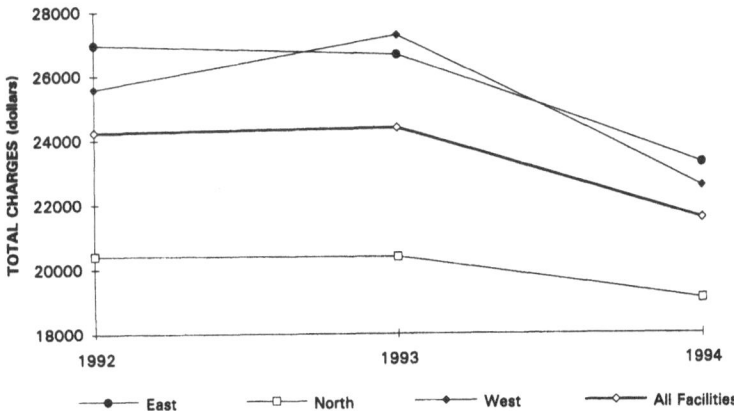

Fig. 3. Total charges (U.S. dollars) for stroke rehabilitation stay

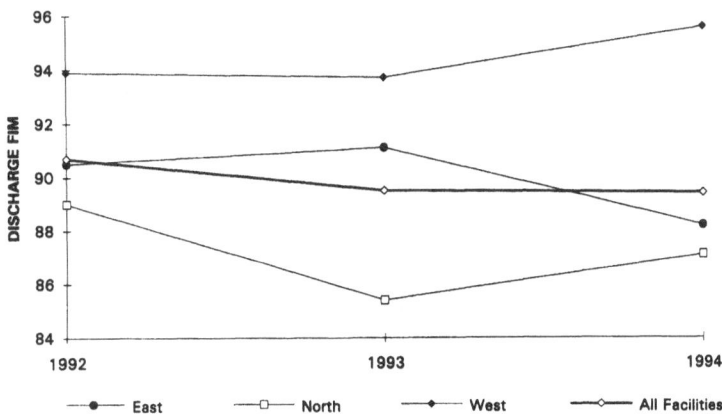

Fig. 4. Functional independence measure (FIM) scores at time of discharge from each facility

Basic administrative and demographic data such as rehabilitation admission dates, length of stay, total charges for rehabilitation services, age, and gender
Basic clinical data, including main diagnoses, date of stroke onset, discharge destination, and FIM levels at admission and discharge

In Fig. 1, patient chronicity in terms of onset–admission interval (OAI) for each facility in each of the 3 years is plotted as the number of days between stroke onset and admission to rehabilitation. OAI dropped markedly at the East facility and less so at the West facility, and at North remained relatively constant during the entire study.

In Fig. 2, the length of stay (LOS) in days for each facility is plotted. The North facility has consistently had the shortest length of stay, about 25 days during the 3 years. The East and West facilities have reduced their LOS during the period of study, approaching the length typical at North. The 10% of patients who stayed fewer than 8 days usually required urgent readmission to the acute care hospital for medical complications.

Figure 3 graphs the total charges in dollars (U.S.) for a stroke rehabilitation stay. The North facility consistently has the lowest cost per admission because its LOS is

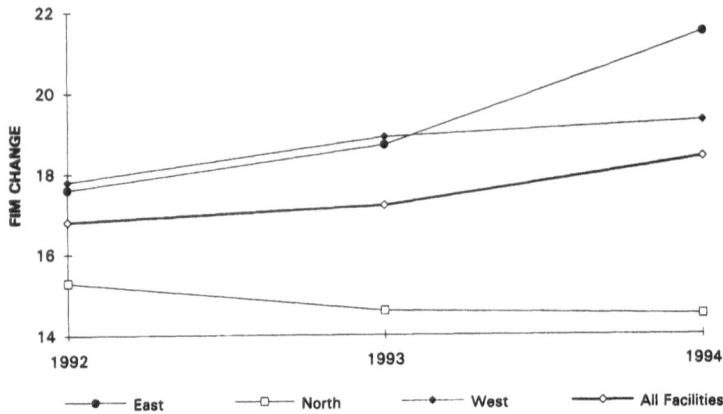

Fig. 5. Change in patient FIM between admission to and discharge from rehabilitation

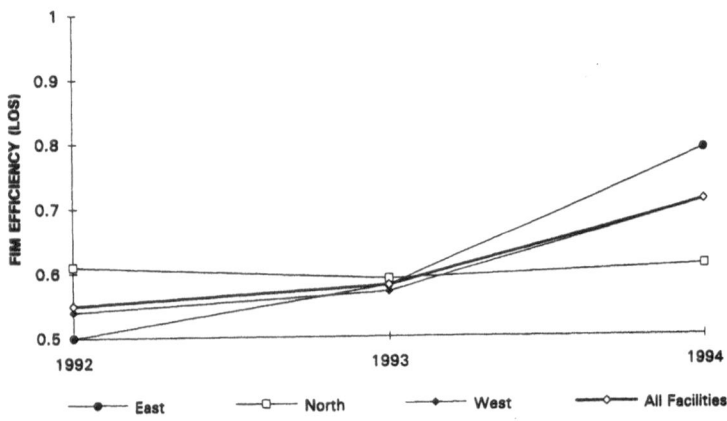

Fig. 6. Program efficiency index, FIM divided by LOS, for each facility

shorter. The East and West facilities both have decreased their total charges per admission during the period of study, which reflects their decreasing average LOS. The East facility recorded slightly higher charges than the West facility in 1994, despite the equal LOS between the two facilities.

In Fig. 4, the discharge FIM scores for a stroke patient are graphed. The North facility discharges its patients at lower FIM levels than do the other facilities, and the West facility discharges its patients at the highest FIM levels. Overall, average discharge FIM scores have not changed across all facilities during the study period.

Figure 5 displays patient functional change in terms of the difference in FIM scores between admission and discharge. The North facility consistently discharges its patients with smaller changes in FIM scores than do the other facilities. The East facility has increased the changes in FIM scores by 3 points. Overall, the changes in FIM scores across all facilities demonstrate small improvements during the study period.

In Fig. 6, an index of program efficiency, FIM-LOS efficiency, was calculated by dividing the FIM change by the LOS for each patient. The North facility has demon-

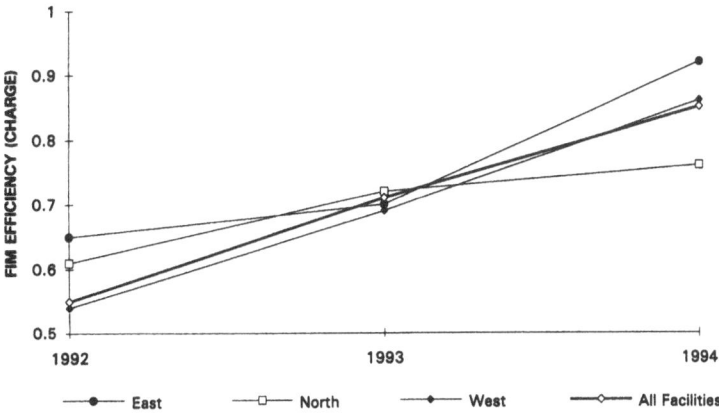

Fig. 7. FIM-charge efficiency, FIM change divided by cost of rehabilitation stay

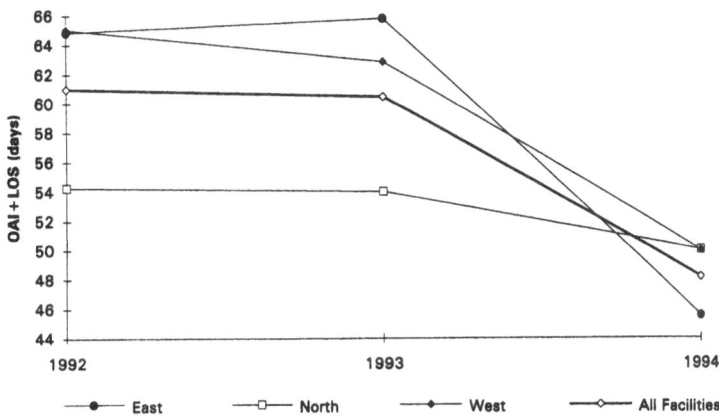

Fig. 8. Total hospitalization time from stroke onset to discharge from rehabilitation

strated a consistent FIM–LOS efficiency per day throughout the entire study period. Both the East and West facilities have demonstrated significant increases in FIM–LOS efficiency during the study period; the East facility has demonstrated a somewhat larger increase.

In Fig. 7, FIM-charge efficiency, reflecting total charges billed during the rehabilitation stay, was calculated by dividing the FIM change per patient by the cost in dollars of the rehabilitation stay. All facilities demonstrated an increase in FIM efficiency per dollar during the study period.

The FIM efficiencies, both per day (Fig. 6) and per dollar (Fig. 7), are explainable. At the North facility, FIM change remained relatively constant throughout the entire study period, as did LOS, thereby resulting in a relatively consistent FIM efficiency. Because rehabilitation cost decreased during the study period, the FIM efficiency per dollar increased. At the West and East facilities, both LOS and rehabilitation cost decreased. During the same period, FIM gain scores were significantly higher and even improved at the East facility. Improvement in FIM gain scores more than offset the longer LOS and the higher costs at the West or East as compared to the North facility.

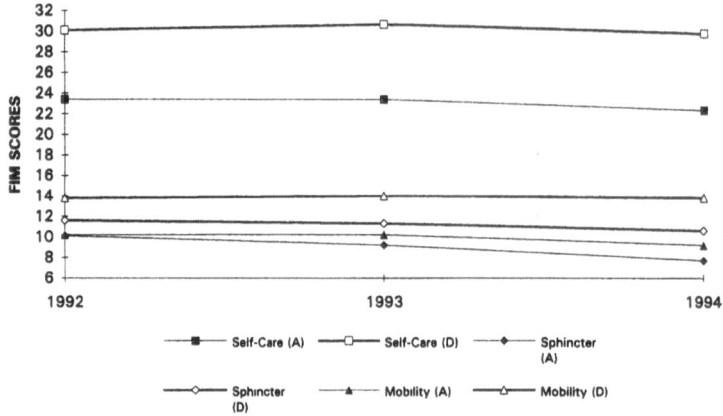

Fig. 9. FIM subscores at admission (A) and discharge (D) for East facility patients during 1992–1994

Figure 8 portrays total hospitalization time from onset of stroke to discharge from the rehabilitation stay, estimated by adding the onset–admission interval (OAI) to the length of rehabilitation stay (LOS). The East and West facilities demonstrated marked decreases in total length of hospitalization, especially between 1993 and 1994; the North facility decreased the total length of hospitalization at a slower pace.

Figure 9 shows admission and discharge FIM subscores of self-care, mobility, and sphincter function in patients who received their inpatient rehabilitation care at the East facility. Average admission function decreased slightly in each of these domains, but discharge function remained constant, during the 3 years.

Discussion

Nationwide Trends

The trends toward shorter rehabilitation LOS experienced in New Jersey (see Fig. 2) reflect broader movements across the United States toward shorter inpatient stays in rehabilitation hospitals and units. The Uniform Data System for Medical Rehabilitation (UDSMR) has published data showing substantial reductions in average rehabilitation hospital LOS in its very large sample [19]. Nationwide LOS declined to 26 days in its sample of just under 40000 such patients in 1993.

The trend toward shorter rehabilitation LOS started in the western United States at least 15–20 years ago, as third-party payers began to look at ways to shave costs. More recently, insurers have begun to develop managed, capitated systems. In these systems, payment is on a per-person basis regardless of services provided, thus providing a potent incentive to provide less costly services. As a consequence, the health care industry in the United States has developed less costly ways to provide rehabilitation services. Large numbers of subacute rehabilitation facilities and nursing home-based rehabilitation programs have recently been developed throughout the country. The northeastern region of the United States has lagged behind this trend. The same pressures have begun to affect Kessler, as reflected in the year-by-year changes we have presented. New Jersey, however, has not yet experienced the full force of the change to capitated and managed health care systems.

The trend toward shorter intervals between stroke onset and rehabilitation admission (OAI) similarly reflects the broader trend toward increasing the brevity of hospital stays. These pressures stem from managed care and the advent of Medicare's prospective payment system (PPS) based on diagnosis-related groups (DRGs) in the early 1980s. Medicare in particular, the largest payer for stroke rehabilitation services, found that the DRG-based prospective payment was effective in slowing the rate of increase of hospital care costs, but not in actually reducing or truly controlling medical costs overall. Rehabilitation hospitals have fortunately been exempt from this prospective payment system and have been paid on a modified cost-per-case basis up to certain limits. Federal agencies have proposed ending this exemption for medical rehabilitation hospitals, but a satisfactory alternative has not yet been developed.

The DRG system, by paying the same amount regardless of LOS, gives acute hospitals a major financial incentive to discharge patients quickly. An early discharge to a rehabilitation hospital can save an acute hospital a great deal of money. The UDSMR reports that the average interval between stroke and rehabilitation admission declined from 22–20 to 19 days between 1991 and 1993. The trend toward shorter OAI is found in the Kessler data as well.

How Short a Stay in Rehabilitation?

How much can patient stays in inpatient rehabilitation be shortened without adversely affecting patient outcomes? We do not know the answer, but we do have data and knowledge that bear on this important question.

UDSMR data report that functional outcomes and gain nationwide were more or less maintained for their stroke sample for 1991, 1992, and 1993:

Average FIM total scores at admission averaged 62.1, 62.0, and 62.6
Average FIM total scores at discharge averaged 87.0, 85.9, and 86.5
Gain scores were 24.9, 23.9, and 23.9
LOS was 32, 28, and 26

The great decline in LOS between 1991 and 1992 was associated with more than doubling the number of participating hospitals (from 108 to 256). While the substantial decline (of 4 days) in LOS between 1991 and 1992 was associated with a 1-point decline in average FIM gain, the further decline in LOS from 28 to 26 days did not affect FIM gain.

The UDSMR has documented improvements in FIM–LOS efficiency between 1990 and 1993. Kessler's figures similarly show improvements. The changes in FIM scores recorded by the East facility (see Fig. 9) are of particular interest. Admission FIM subscores either remained unchanged or decreased between 1992 and 1994. Despite declining LOS during these years, discharge FIM remained relatively constant. Thus, LOS was reduced without deterioration in patient function.

These is reason to believe that the shortening of LOS cannot go on indefinitely without negatively affecting gains in patient function. It is known that longer stays are associated with greater average patient functional gain between admission and discharge in rehabilitation. This relationship is reflected in the positive "LOS efficiency" and "FIM gain per week" figures documented by the UDSMR. On the other hand, it is quite conceivable that LOS can be shortened further without significant effect on long-term outcomes, if programs reorganize to meet this objective. We know of hospital-based rehabilitation facilities that report lengths of stay averaging 21 days or less for stroke patients.

To reduce LOS, precautions must be observed to ensure that a stroke survivor is discharged safely to home. For example (Fig. 4), the North facility discharged its patients home at lower levels of function until 1994. Discharges at lower levels of function are appropriate when the team is able to recruit the family to supervise or assist the patient in a safe manner, thus allowing a quicker transition to home. The West facility, on the other hand, discharged its stroke survivors home at a higher level of function than the other faciltes. Such longer stays are appropriate when patients have fewer family resources, but longer stays can also indicate inefficiency or more accommodating sources of payment. If the latter is true, the LOS may be reduced further to match the discharge functional levels of the North and East facilities.

Reduction in LOS is also possible by addressing the organization of treatment services during the week. During the years studied, stroke patients were admitted to Kessler facilities only on weekdays, from Monday to Friday, although only 14% of admissions were on Monday with the remainder spread evenly throughout the week. Discharges were also primarily during the 5-day workweek, with the West and East facilities discharging only 5% of patients on a Monday and another 5% on Saturday or Sunday. North discharges were somewhat more even, with 10% on Monday and another 10% over the weekend. LOS showed a specific pattern, with one-quarter of patients discharged on the same day of the week on which they had been admitted; particular concentrations in LOS occurred at 21, 28, and 35 days. Kessler now is increasing therapy services on the weekends and planning specific discharge dates within the first week of admission to allow discharge of patients at the earliest possible day. Furthermore, 10% of our stroke patients are discharged in fewer than 8 days, most often to return to the acute care hospital for sudden medical problems. Of these, one-third are discharged on a Friday; this would suggest either that there are more medical problems on Friday (unlikely) or that acute problems are more often handled in the rehabilitation facility on other days of the week, rather than relying on transfer to an acute care facility.

We believe that the trend of shorter OAIs can and should continue until OAIs have reached 7 to 10 days. Likewise, we fully expect that the trends toward shorter lengths of stay at Kessler will continue. To accomplish appropriate but still earlier discharges, acute and rehabilitation hospitals are currently developing *critical pathways* or *clinical paths*. These are statements of critical processes and objectives to be met on a day-to-day basis to enable patients in a diagnostic group to be discharged in a specified period of time. So long as needed support from family, outpatient clinics, and visiting nurse and home therapy programs is available, stroke survivors should be able to return to the community even faster, with decreased rehabilitation costs, and without significant adverse affects on patient functioning, family stress, or patient health. Family members will need to be fully involved in the rehabilitation process at its very inception so that they may take responsibility of the care of the stroke survivor at increasingly earlier times. At the same time, stringent studies are required to monitor the effects of ever-decreasing lengths of stay.

Conclusion

A system for functional evaluation and treatment of stroke survivors in a group of rehabilitation hospitals in New Jersey (United States) has been described. Trends in length of stay and function outcomes have been presented for three rehabilitation facilities and contrasted with national trends in the 1990s.

Ever-increasing pressure has been placed on health care providers to decrease the cost of rehabilitation. Rehabilitation professionals must nonetheless address continuing needs to maximize the function and ensure the safety of stroke survivors. To do this, rehabilitation professionals need to develop creative ways to facilitate recovery and teach compensatory strategies earlier and during shorter timeframes. Stroke survivors will become more dependent on less intensive modes of service provision, such as subacute rehabilitation facilities, home therapy services, nursing home-based rehabilitation facilities, and outpatient services. By integrating all these features into its program, institutions such as the Kessler Institute can continue to provide high-quality, effective rehabilitation to its patients while meeting demands of the government and the insurance industry to curb the growth of rehabilitation and disability-related costs.

References

1. Dombovy ML, Sandok BA, Basford JA (1986) Rehabilitation for stroke: a review. Stroke 17(3):363–369
2. Lehmann JF, DeLateur BJ, Fowler RS, et al (1975) Stroke rehabilitation: outcome and prediction. Arch Phys Med Rehabil 56:383–389
3. Matcher DB, Duncan PW (1994) Cost of stroke. Stroke: Clinical Updates 5(3):9–12
4. Johnston MV, Zorowitz RD, Nash B (1994) Family help available. Top Geriatr Rehabil 9(3):38–53
5. Johnston MV, Kirshblum S, Zorowitz RD, Shiflett SC (1992) Prediction of outcomes following rehabilitation of stroke patients. NeuroRehabilitation 2(4):71–96
6. Harbison JW (1992) Ticlopidine versus aspirin for the prevention of recurrent stroke. Stroke 23:1723–1727
7. Bellavance A (1993) Efficacy of ticlopidine and aspirin for prevention of reversible cerebrovascular ischemic events: the ticlopidine aspirin study. Stroke 24:1452–1457
8. Grotta JC, Norris JW, Kamm B (1992) Prevention of stroke with ticlopidine: who benefits most? Neurology 42(1):111–115
9. Acheson J, Danta G, Hutchinson EC (1969) Controlled trial of dipyridamole in cerebral vascular disease. Br Med J 1:614–615
10. The American-Canadian Cooperative Study Group (1985) Persantine aspirin trial in cerebral ischemia. Part II: Endpoint results. Stroke 16:406–415
11. Bowton DL, Stump DA, Prough DS, Toole JF, Lefkowitz DS, Coker L (1989) Pentoxifylline increases cerebral blood flow in patients with cerebrovascular disease. Stroke 20:1662–1666
12. Irie K, Yamaguchi T, Minematus K, Omae T (1993) The j-curve phenomenon in stroke recurrence. Stroke 24:1844–1849
13. Bromfield EB, Reding MB (1988) Relative risk of deep venous thrombosis or pulmonary embolism post-stroke based upon ambulatory status. J Neuro Rehabil 2(2):51–56
14. Linsenmeyer TA, Zorowitz RD (1992) Urodynamic findings of patients with urinary incontinence following cerebrovascular accident. NeuroRehabilitation 2(4):23–26
15. Veis SL, Logemann JA (1985) Swallowing disorders in persons with cerebrovascular accident. Arch Phys Med Rehabil 66(6):372–375
16. Horner J, Massey EW, Riski JE, Lathrop DL, Chase KN (1988) Aspiration following stroke: clinical correlates and outcome. Neurology 38:1359–1362
17. Horner J, Massey EW (1988) Silent aspiration following stroke. Neurology 38:317–319
18. Granger CV, Cotter AC, Hamilton BB, Fielder RC (1993) Functional assessment scales: a study of persons after stroke. Arch Phys Med Rehabil 74:133–138
19. Granger CV, Ottenbacher KJ, Fiedler RC (1993) The Uniform Data System for Medical Rehabilitation: report of first admissions for 1993. Am J Phys Med Rehabil 74(1):62–66

The Functional Independence Measure: A Measurement of Disability and Medical Rehabilitation

Roger C. Fiedler and Carl V. Granger[1]

Summary. Measuring outcomes in medical rehabilitation must begin with an under-standing of what is to be measured, and this understanding must be grounded in theory and connected to a comprehensive model for meeting the needs of the patient. Measurement tools for outcomes must then be designed and tested with respect to their purpose, practicality, construction, standardization, reliability, and validity. This chapter proposes a conceptual model called Challenges to the Quality of Daily Living that is based on the work of Abraham Maslow. The model describes the goal of fulfillment as achieving a balance between one's choices, options, and expectations on the one hand (functional opportunities), with one's physical, cognitive, and emotional constraints (functional demands/barriers) on the other. While these opportunities and demands are not directly measurable in qualitative or quantitative terms, the underlying factors supporting or forming barriers to health and function are measur-able. The Functional Independence Measure (FIM) and the Uniform Data System for Medical Rehabilitation (UDSMR) are examined from the perspectives described above, and are found to provide practical measurement for patients undergoing medical rehabilitation for conditions that render them dependent on others for assis-tance in activities of daily living. The FIM has been shown to be reliable, valid, feasible, practical, and sensitive to clinical change in functional independence at admission, discharge, and follow-up. Use of the FIM and the UDSMR characterizes disability and change in severity through the use of a uniform language, and has important implica-tions for national and international exchange of comparable information concerning outcomes.

Introduction

The recent emphasis on medical rehabilitation outcomes has highlighted the need to examine the scales and measures currently used to determine the outcomes of patient care management. Several recent publications have detailed clear plans and proce-dures for evaluating such scales and measures to ensure reliable and valid outcome assessments. Johnston et al. [1] have provided a standardized set of procedures for

[1]Center for Functional Assessment Research, Department of Rehabilitation Medicine, School of Medicine and Biomedical Sciences, State University of New York at Buffalo, Buffalo, NY 14214, USA

examining the use and value of medical rehabilitation scales. They state that the key questions when designing and/or evaluating a scale are identifying its purpose, determining its practicality for clinical use, determining if the items and scoring system(s) are acceptable and useful, determining the standardization of procedures for administration and scoring, and testing whether the scale is reliable and valid. Scales failing to meet these standards may be judged to be suspect in benefits to patients [2], as they may not be useful indicators of medical rehabilitation outcomes. All medical rehabilitation scales should be examined with this set of standards in mind to judge their value to the profession and the patients.

The Functional Independence Measure (FIM) is an example of one such scale that is grounded in good clinical theory and was clearly designed to provide an indicator of disability independent of a patient's impairment. Designed by a multidisciplinary clinical task force, it consists of 18 items, each rated on a seven-level scale from (1) indicating *complete functional dependence* to (7) indicating *complete functional independence*. It is quickly and easily administered by any trained clinician, has a clearly established and standardized administration protocol, and has been extensively tested for reliability and validity. Thus, the FIM meets all the standards set by Johnston et al. The FIM therefore is an ideal indicator of medical rehabilitation outcomes because it meets all the proper measurement standard. Although published as unique to medical rehabilitation, such standards are in fact common to all professions in which measurement tools are used as indicators of outcomes.

Because the FIM has received such intensive scrutiny by both clinical and psychometric (or clinometric) experts during the past 8 years, it serves as a useful example of how such an examination of measurement standards should proceed. It is important to note that the process of examining the FIM according to the standards just outlined is not presented in its original chronological order here, but in the order that the standards recommend.

What is the Purpose of the FIM?

All measurements and scales should be grounded in a clear theoretical statement of their goals and intent. The FIM was originally constructed by the Task Force in 1987 [3] to be a measure of disability independent of impairment, in keeping with the theoretical conceptualization of the terms of impairment, disability, and handicap as expressed by Nagi [4] and the World Health Organization model [5]. More recently, however, the FIM has been grounded in a new conceptual/theoretical model of medical rehabilitation, described as the Model of Challenges to the Quality of Daily Living, and has found its expression in the diagram displayed in Fig. 1.

Measuring outcomes in medical rehabilitation must begin with an understanding of what is to be measured, and this understanding must be grounded in theory and connected to a comprehensive model for meeting the needs of the patient. One critical problem that has hampered the development of good measurement tools in medical rehabilitation has been the inability of health care professionals to speak a common language. Several conceptual and theoretical models have provided differing definitions of patient impairment, disability, and handicap. To begin the process of comprehensively measuring disability and outcomes in medical rehabilitation, the following operational definition of quality of daily living is offered:

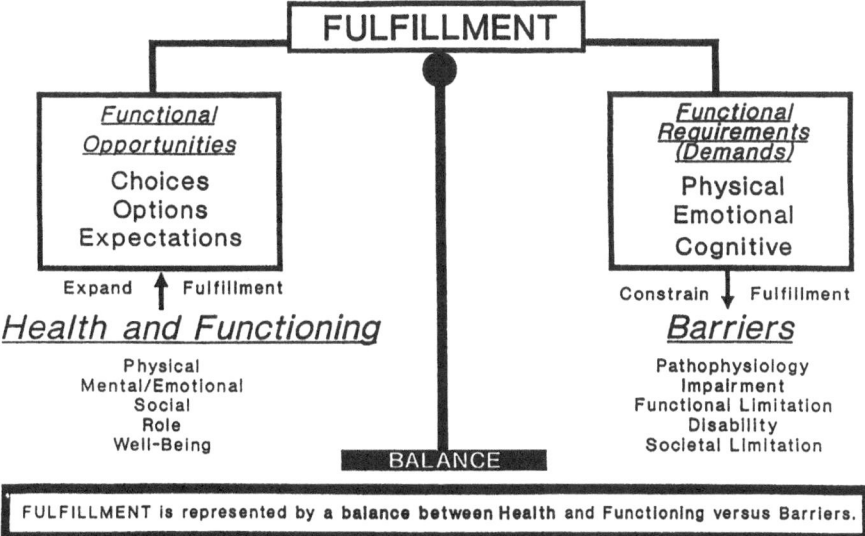

Fig. 1. Challenges to the quality of daily living

Quality of daily living is the ever-changing balance between one's choices, options, and expectations versus the physical, cognitive, and emotional demands of daily living.

With this definition in place, measurement of disability outcomes in medical rehabilitation may be envisioned as shown in Fig. 1. This diagram represents a Model for Challenges to the Quality of Daily Living in anticipation of an integrated science of medical rehabilitation based upon a firm foundation of sound theory and scientific measurement principles. The model (Fig. 1) allows for the development, measurement, and testing of an entirely new organizing and unifying concept for studying disablement and medical rehabilitation and covers a broad range of concerns currently under debate. This model views fulfillment as a result of achieving a balance in life between the functional opportunities available to the individual and the functional requirements or demands placed on the individual.

The Challenges to the Quality of Daily Living model develops from the work of the noted American psychologist, Abraham Maslow. Maslow [6] advanced a new theory of human motivation that challenged some of the orthodox principles of Freudian and Skinnerian psychology. Before Maslow, it had been considered appropriate to control and manipulate employees in the workplace. In the 1960s, Maslow developed the "Eupsychian management" way of thinking to encourage a more humanistic relationship between management and employees. From this, Maslow evolved a hierarchy of needs that would support self-actualization. At the base of his conceptual pyramid lay the physical needs for survival. At progressively higher levels were satisfaction of needs for security, social interaction, and self-esteem. As lower level needs were satisfied, then successively higher levels of need became relatively more important as motivators of behavior. Ultimately, the fully evolved individual would achieve self-actualization, a term that describes the full utilization of human capacities to perceive, feel, learn, acquire skill, exercise intellectual capabilities, create, love—in short, based on self-esteem and respect for others, to grow in competence and ability to live a fulfilling life [6].

Maslow's concepts form the conceptual framework for the study of disability outcomes. Medical rehabilitation is a system of interdisciplinary interventions designed to facilitate fulfillment and the quality of daily living for individuals with disabilities. Rehabilitation needs measurement that can reflect the effectiveness and efficiency of this process. To a large extent, however, fulfillment and quality of daily living are not directly measurable. To account for the challenges to fulfillment and the quality of daily living, one must begin by identifying the factors that determine the opportunities and requirements (demands). Figure 1 proposes that an individual's fulfillment and quality of daily living are a result of striking a balance between functional opportunities (on the left) and functional requirements or demands (on the right). Functional opportunities are expressed as the individual's choices, options, and expectations, while functional requirements are expressed in physical, cognitive, and emotional terms. To achieve fulfillment and to maximize the quality of daily living, there must be a balance between improved opportunities through individual health and functioning (on the left) and the reduction or removal of life's barriers causing constraints (on the right).

This model reflects Maslow's industrial psychological beliefs that health and functioning result when the individual is presented with life's work in the form of barriers and systematically overcomes them. The model further reflects Maslow's hierarchical beliefs by viewing the disabled individual as meeting progressively higher needs of function through the work of medical rehabilitation. The field of medical rehabilitation recognizes the need for balance between functional demands and functional opportunities, progressively presenting both the demands and the ways to achieve the opportunities to the patient in the form of challenges to the quality of daily living, and moving up the hierarchy from the basic physical needs to the satisfaction for security, social interaction, and self-esteem. The ultimate goal of medical rehabilitation then becomes, in Maslow's terms, self-actualization, the full utilization of the human capacities to perceive, feel, create, and love, in the form of fulfillment through the everyday efforts to challenge barriers and overcome them.

Figure 1 includes several measurable factors that serve as domains of health and functioning (on the left), such as physical, mental/emotional, social, role performance, and subjective well-being, while measurable barriers (on the right) include pathophysiology, impairment, functional limitation, disability, and societal limitation.

This unifying model for medical rehabilitation fits well with existing theoretical frameworks across the many disciplines involved in medical rehabilitation (e.g., the Open Systems Theory models of von Bertalanffy [7] and Kielhofner and Burke [8]) of hierarchical structures and expanding and constraining relationships between levels of the hierarchy, and provides an organizing conceptual framework for measuring disability across disciplines. The model recognizes that functional opportunities and requirements which serve as the challenges to the quality of daily living are not directly measurable, but that the factors which determine the opportunities and requirements are subject to description and measurement.

The Model of Challenges to the Quality of Daily Living (Fig. 1) suggests that fulfillment results from a balance between the functional opportunities to expand health and functioning through choices, options, and expectations while at the same time overcoming the challenges of functional barriers in the form of physical, emotional, and cognitive demands that constrain function. It is clear that examination of such complexity is not easily achieved through current medical rehabilitation measures, but the factors determining the opportunities and requirements or demands are subject to description and measurement. One goal of developing such a model is translating concepts into measurement systems and then implementing those systems into clinical practice through research.

To determine how well a conceptual theoretical model fits the field of medical rehabilitation, the model must be judged on comprehensiveness while subject to the principles of good measurement, and its practicality in implementation and must be rigorously tested by patients, clinicians, administrators, and researchers. The proposed model is quite comprehensive, allowing a multidisciplinary approach to medical rehabilitation. Translating the model into measurement and implementing it into the clinical arena to be judged by patients and clinicians has begun with the use of the Functional Independence Measure (FIM) at the Uniform Data System for Medical Rehabilitation (UDSMR) at the State University of New York at Buffalo.

The test of the ability of the FIM to meet the measurement standards of Johnston et al. moves to the next step by determining whether the scale has practical clinical use. The UDSMR has resulted in the use of the FIM in more than 60% of medical rehabilitation facilities across the United States and has moved the FIM from continental use to international use by translations into Australian, Canadian, French, German, Italian, Japanese, Portuguese, Spanish, and Swedish versions. This broad base of clinical use has allowed the FIM to be examined from a wide variety of perspectives and in a wide variety of locations around the world. Some of the results of this exposure are described here.

Is the Scale Practical for Clinical Use?

With all other factors being equal, most clinicians would prefer to use shorter rather than longer scales to assess their patients. The FIM is an easy scale to administer, with a minimum data set of 18 items, each rated on a seven-level scale. The ease of administration of the FIM, and its design by a task force of medical rehabilitation experts to be discipline free, make it especially practical to use by any trained clinician.

One criterion for judging whether a scale is practical for clinical use is to test it in clinical environments for face validity, the extent to which clinicians agree that the scale measures what it was designed to measure. As the FIM has been used in more than 60% of U.S. medical rehabilitation facilities and has been translated into several languages for use internationally, the FIM may be said to have outstanding face validity. Progressive development of the FIM into such widespread use has resulted in part from its practicality, its ease of use, and its face validity. Further, the FIM has been incorporated into the UDSMR, which has a large number of subscribing facilities. The next section describes some of the design and activities of the UDSMR.

What is the UDSMR?

The UDSMR is a not-for-profit organization developed and managed under the auspices of the Center for Functional Assessment Research, Department of Rehabilitation

Medicine, School of Medicine and Biomedical Sciences, at the State University of New York at Buffalo. The UDSMR was established in 1987 and developed with grant support from the U.S. Department of Education, National Institute of Disability and Rehabilitation Research (grant number G008435062, entitled Development of a Uniform National Data System for Medical Rehabilitation, a field-initiated project directed by C.V. Granger, M.D., and B.B. Hamilton, M.D., Ph.D.). Sponsoring, cooperating, and endorsing organizations included the American Congress of Rehabilitation Medicine, American Academy of Physical Medicine and Rehabilitation, American Physical Therapy Association, American Occupational Therapy Association, American Speech, Language and Hearing Association, Association of Rehabilitation Nurses, National Association of Rehabilitation Facilities, Commission on Accreditation of Rehabilitation Facilities, American Hospital Association (Section for Rehabilitation Hospitals and Programs), National Association of Research and Training Centers, American Spinal Injury Association, National Head Injury Foundation, and National Easter Seals Society. Today, support for UDSMR comes from the School of Medicine and Biomedical Sciences, research grants, and fees from Data Management Service subscriptions and training.

The UDSMR is managed by the director and resources of the Center for Functional Assessment Research of the Department of Rehabilitation Medicine with approval of the Executive Board representing the State University of New York at Buffalo and with the advice of a National Advisory Committee.

Why Was the UDSMR Developed?

At the annual meetings of the American Congress of Rehabilitation Medicine and the American Academy of Physical Medicine and Rehabilitation in November 1983, a joint task force was appointed to develop a methodology for satisfying a long-standing need to document severity of patient disability and the outcomes of medical rehabilitation. At that time, there had been no *uniform* way to describe and communicate about disability.

What Does the UDSMR Do?

The mission of the UDSMR includes the following:

1. To establish and maintain a uniform language and definitions for communicating about disability and rehabilitation outcome. The elements are the dataset (descriptors), the database (aggregate of data on patients), data management (quality control and reporting), and other elements of a comprehensive data system

2. To collect data, provide information, and foster research that will uniformly characterize disability and change in severity through use of uniform language, definitions, and measurements

3. To establish and maintain a common data collection and reporting process that the majority of rehabilitation facilities can use and find beneficial for comparing and evaluating service outcomes

The data for UDSMR are based upon a minimum data aggregate composed of demographic, diagnostic, functional, and charge information. UDSMR provides streamlined data collection forms, software, and standardized directions allowing facilities to uniformly document, monitor, and compare outcomes of rehabilitated patients. Data are forwarded quarterly to the UDSMR for analysis and reporting back to participating facilities, providing confidential facility and aggregate regional and national data. A Guide for the Uniform Data Set for Medical Rehabilitation [3], the main form of standardization, is periodically updated. An instrument for measurement of disability in children, called the WeeFIM, has been developed and tested. A reporting system for WeeFIM is being developed that allows the facility to accumulate and compare repeated patient assessments over time. A UDSMR newsletter is distributed to about 4500 addresses worldwide; national and international training sessions are conducted, and publications are produced to promote uniformity in the use of the dataset and to help improve the effectiveness and efficiency of the medical rehabilitation process.

A number of uniform descriptors and calculations, offered to UDSMR subscribers for comparative purposes [9,10].

Measurement of Efficiency

Length of Stay: Average change in FIM per day of rehabilitation hospital stay is calculated by subtracting admission FIM from discharge FIM and then dividing by length of stay in days. This is a crude but useful measure of care efficiency; the higher the number, the greater the efficiency. The advantage of using length of stay (LOS) efficiency is that variation in charges between regions is avoided. LOS efficiency by impairment group is probably the most reliable and useful means of assessing and comparing care efficiency.

Charges: Average change in FIM per $1000 charge is calculated by subtracting admission FIM from discharge FIM, then dividing the gain by charges (in dollars), multiplied by 1000. Multiplying by 1000 makes the numbers close to 1, which is more easily understood. This is a more conventional expression of "cost" efficiency; the higher the number, the higher the efficiency. That is, the higher the benefit (gain) and the lower the "cost" (charge), the more efficient the care process. However, the same considerations for interpretation must be applied to efficiency as to charges. Region, case mix, and other variables do influence charge efficiency. Charge efficiency by impairment group is reported.

Discharge Destination

Community discharge is discharge to home, board and care, or transitional living. Long-term care discharge is to intermediate care, a skilled nursing facility, or a chronic care hospital. Preparing patients for independent living in the community is a major rehabilitation objective. There is generally a correlation between achieving higher levels of function during rehabilitation (e.g., higher FIM) and a greater percentage of patients living independently in the community. A FIM score of about 80 or greater is required for patients returning successfully to care of a household member, or 100 or better if the patient lives alone. Some communities and families are more capable of providing independent living conditions than others, however, and this will influence the percentage of patients going to the community.

Program Evaluation and Performance Index

The Program Evaluation Model provides an example of how a facility may compare its performance in five program objective areas with expected performance using a format similar to that suggested by the Commission on Accreditation of Rehabilitation Facilities (CARF).

The five program objectives in the model are:

1. Achieving a high percentage of patients discharged to independent living in the community
2. Achieving a high effectiveness (FIM gain from admission to discharge)
3. Serving and benefiting more severely disabled individuals
4. Minimizing rehabilitation length of stay
5. Minimizing the total charges for the rehabilitation length of stay

The Performance Index is a weighted score of these measures comparing a given facility with the regional and national averages. A score greater than 100 means that a facility has a higher performance index compared with the region or national group; a score lower than 100 means a lower performance index. The rank ordering of facilities by Performance Index, developed for each impairment group, gives an indication where a given facility stands, compared with all others.

What is the Current Status of the UDSMR?

Cumulative admission–discharge patient records (plus more than 30% follow-up) have grown to more than 600 000 at the end of 1994. Subscribing facilities receive quarterly standard reports showing all patients for the past rolling 12 months, first admissions only for the past rolling 12 months, and first admissions for the past 3 months. Multifacility corporate reports and other special reports are provided. There are more than 500 U.S. facility subscribers (about 60% of all U.S. rehabilitation facilities) plus subscribing facilities in Canada, Australia, and Japan. The UDSMR will continue to establish and maintain fundamental, uniform definitions and measures of disability and care outcomes for the field of medical rehabilitation for use with adults and children in hospitals, outpatient, and alternative care settings. Functional assessment research initiatives will continue to advance the care processes and to improve rehabilitation outcomes for persons with disability.

How was the Scale Constructed?

The key element of the UDSMR is the FIM, a measure of disability. The FIM is applicable to patients of all impairment types under the care of rehabilitation inpatient facilities and consists of 13 motor and 5 cognitive items measured on an ordinal seven-level scale. The FIM is discipline free and is a quickly administered, minimal descriptor of a patient's level of functioning. The FIM was designed to provide uniformity in terminology and allow clinicians and researchers to track patients from the initiation of a treatment intervention through discharge and follow-up.

The FIM measures a patient's performance of basic activities of daily living using 18 items within six subscales of self-care (eating, grooming, bathing, dressing upper and lower body, and toileting), sphincter control (bladder and bowel management), mobility (transfers to bed/chair/wheelchair, toilet, and tub/shower), locomotion (walking/wheeling and stair climbing), communication (comprehension and expression), and social cognition (social interaction, memory, and problem-solving). The seven levels of performance reflect the extent to which the activities are performed independently or require the help of another person. A higher score means that the person is more independent. A score on the FIM is a way of representing the "burden of care" or cost of disability in terms of the amount of effort needed from another person and the costs in terms of consumption of social and economic resources.

The multiplicity of functional status outcome scales used in different rehabilitation hospitals is believed to have been contributing to confusion regarding outcomes of medical rehabilitation. The FIM was developed to offer the field a uniform method for describing the severity of disability and the functional outcomes of medical rehabilitation.

Development of the FIM and the UDSMR were unique in that they evolved through a process of national consensus followed by a systematic procedure of evaluation. After reviewing 36 published and unpublished functional assessment instruments, the challenge was to select the most common and useful functional assessment items and to decide on an appropriate rating scale that would permit most rehabilitation clinicians to assess severity of disability in a uniform and reliable manner. Investigation was carried out in three phases: pilot, trial, and implementation. The pilot was completed in the spring of 1985, using 11 facilities and 110 patients to determine the face validity and ease of administration. The intent of the trial, completed in 1986, was to assess interrater reliability, validity, precision, and time to administer the data set. Data for the trial were obtained at admission, discharge and, when feasible, follow-up after discharge in 25 facilities nationwide on 250 patients using 891 clinician assessments [11].

Implementation phase evaluation in 18 facilities with 303 patients in 1987 finalized the seven-level scale, revised from the original four-level scale, and confirmed the face validity and precision findings of the trial. Interrater reliability improved (FIM total score intraclass correlation reached .95), with FIM learning time averaging about an hour and FIM administration time averaging about a half-hour.

The principal method for clinician training was the printed *Guide for the Uniform Data Set for Medical Rehabilitation* [3]. Standardization of understanding and use of the FIM, a top priority, is being accomplished through revisions of the Guide (latest version, 4.0, March 1993) to clarify language and expand definitions of terms. More than 5000 clinicians have been trained through formal and informal training workshops, and training videotapes have been distributed. The quarterly newsletter (*UDSMR UPDATE*) is mailed to about 4500 addresses worldwide to advise users on rating patients and use of the data. There is a program of credentialing reliability of FIM raters by means of an examination that tests understanding of the FIM definitions. A clinician must attain a grade of 80% to pass, and a facility must have 80% of its clinicians pass the test, as well as having its data pass a technical review, for its data to be included in the regional and national aggregations.

FIM has utility features of comprehensiveness, effectiveness, efficiency, comparability, and predictability. Comprehensiveness of the FIM is demonstrated by its use as a principal gauge of the major functional and behavioral activities that represent "burden of care." Effectiveness is demonstrated through changes in the FIM scores that track the status of a person's disability in the direction sought by the program. Efficiency is demonstrated by an analysis of the relationships between the cost and duration of a program and the person's pre- and postrehabilitation levels of functional status. Comparability is facilitated because outcomes of programs are described in a uniform manner. Predictability allows facility administrators and clinicians to use the compiled database to predict which persons are best served by the program, the kinds and amounts of services needed, and the likelihood of obtaining the desired results. The major benefit is facilitation of effectiveness and efficiency of rehabilitation services. This is useful to rehabilitation providers, policy makers and planners, with ultimate benefit to the patients, their families, and the community.

The kinds of questions that the scale may be expected to help answer depend on how the scale is classified: (1) discriminative, (2) predictive, or (3) evaluative. For example, the FIM helps to quantify disability to discriminate between classes of subjects with respect to severity of disability; it helps to predict discharge to living in the community rather than in a nursing home or to predict the cost of maintaining a patient with disability if there is no further improvement; and it is evaluative, permitting one to detect clinically important change when it occurs. Therefore, the FIM contributes to answering all three questions. Because the FIM is a reliable and valid measure of disability, it may be combined with other data elements to investigate and understand how to improve the effectiveness and efficiency of medical rehabilitation.

In determining how a scale is constructed, rigorous psychometric examination of its content becomes a key concern. Although the FIM was constructed through the efforts of a task force designed to create a uniform measure of disability that was easy to use, discipline free, and applicable across a wide variety of impairments and settings, the FIM has been extensively tested through psychometric studies of its content. Recent studies using Rasch analyses [12,13] have confirmed that the FIM measures both motor and cognitive functioning. Figure 2 shows the FIM items and subscales, with the first 13 items representing the motor functioning areas of self-care, sphincter control, mobility, and locomotion. The last 5 items represent cognitive functioning in the areas of communication and social cognition. The FIM is one of the few scales in the field of medical rehabilitation that has received extensive evaluation by measurement experts. Additional information about its measurement properties with regard to reliability and validity using both raw scores and Rasch measures is discussed next.

There has been considerable discussion about the ordinal level of the FIM items, and further debate in the literature about the issue of whether the FIM total scores represent an ordinal or an interval level scale. The contribution of Rasch studies [12,14] has been to convert the raw scores for FIM motor and FIM cognitive scales to interval-level Rasch measures using a conversion table. Thus, Table 1 shows the conversion figures developed by Linacre (personal communication, 1992) for changing raw scores to interval-level measures.

Is the Scale Standardized?

The FIM is a standardized scale with guides available from the UDSMR. FIM guides provide clear details about scoring each item, and UDSMR newsletters provide additional coding tips on the use of the FIM items in unusual cases. One of the most important recent advances in the use of the FIM by UDSMR subscribers has been the development of FIM software with considerable flexibility for both clinical and research purposes. The FIMware which is now available provides interactive directions for scoring the FIM. The software is designed in such a way as to prevent the user from

————————————————————————————————▶

Fig. 2. The Functional Independence Measure (FIM)

	7 Complete Independence (Timely, Safely) 6 Modified Independence (Device)	NO HELPER

L E V E L S	Modified Dependence
	   5 Supervision
	   4 Minimal Assist (Subject = 75% +)
	   3 Moderate Assist (Subject = 50% +)
	
	Complete Dependence
	   2 Maximal Assist (Subject = 25% +)
	   1 Total Assist (Subject = 0% +)
		HELPER

	ADMIT	DISCHG	FOL-UP
Self-Care A. Eating B. Grooming C. Bathing D. Dressing - Upper Body E. Dressing - Lower Body F. Toileting	☐☐☐☐☐☐	☐☐☐☐☐☐	☐☐☐☐☐☐
Sphincter Control G. Bladder Management H. Bowel Management	☐☐	☐☐	☐☐
Transfers I. Bed, Chair, Wheelchair J. Toilet K. Tub, Shower	☐☐☐	☐☐☐	☐☐☐
Locomotion L. Walk/wheelchair M. Stairs	Walk/Wheelchair/Both ☐☐ ☐	Walk/Wheelchair/Both ☐☐ ☐	Walk/Wheelchair/Both ☐☐ ☐
Motor Subtotal Score	☐	☐	☐
Communication N. Comprehension O. Expression	Auditory/Visual/Both ☐ Vocal/Non-vocal/Both ☐	Auditory/Visual/Both ☐ Vocal/Non-vocal/Both ☐	Auditory/Visual/Both ☐ Vocal/Non-vocal/Both ☐
Social Cognition P. Social Interaction Q. Problem Solving R. Memory	☐☐☐	☐☐☐	☐☐☐
Cognitive Subtotal Score	☐	☐	☐
Total FIM	☐	☐	☐

NOTE: Leave no blanks; enter 1 if patient not testable due to risk

Table 1. Expected item scores corresponding to individual FIM scores for motor and cognitive Functional Independence Measure (FIM) scales.

FIM Score	A	B	C	D	E	F	G	H	I	J	K	L	M	0–100 Meas	S.E.
13	1	1	1	1	1	1	1	1	1	1	1	1	1	0	10
14	2	1	1	1	1	1	1	1	1	1	1	1	1	10	10
15	2	2	1	1	1	1	1	1	1	1	1	1	1	16	7
16	2	2	1	1	1	1	1	2	1	1	1	1	1	20	5
17	2	2	1	1	1	1	2	2	1	1	1	1	1	22	5
18	2	2	1	2	1	1	2	2	1	1	1	1	1	24	4
19	3	2	1	2	1	1	2	2	1	1	1	1	1	26	4
20	3	2	1	2	1	1	2	2	2	1	1	1	1	27	4
21	3	2	1	2	1	2	2	2	2	1	1	1	1	28	4
22	3	2	1	2	1	2	2	2	2	2	1	1	1	29	3
23	3	3	1	2	1	2	2	2	2	2	1	1	1	30	3
24	3	3	2	2	1	2	2	2	2	2	1	1	1	31	3
25	3	3	2	2	2	2	2	2	2	2	1	1	1	32	3
26	4	3	2	2	2	2	2	2	2	2	1	1	1	33	3
27	4	3	2	2	2	2	2	3	2	2	1	1	1	34	3
28	4	3	2	2	2	2	2	3	2	2	1	2	1	35	3
29	4	3	2	2	2	2	3	3	2	2	1	2	1	35	3
30	4	3	2	3	2	2	3	3	2	2	1	2	1	36	3
31	4	4	2	3	2	2	3	3	2	2	1	2	1	37	3
32	4	4	2	3	2	2	3	3	2	2	2	2	1	37	3
33	5	4	2	3	2	2	3	3	2	2	2	2	1	38	3
34	5	4	2	3	2	2	3	3	3	2	2	2	1	39	2
35	5	4	2	3	2	2	3	4	3	2	2	2	1	39	2
36	5	4	2	3	2	3	3	4	3	2	2	2	1	40	2
37	5	4	2	3	2	3	4	4	3	2	2	2	1	40	2
38	5	4	2	4	2	3	4	4	3	2	2	2	1	41	2
39	5	4	2	4	2	3	4	4	3	3	2	2	1	42	2
40	5	4	3	4	2	3	4	4	3	3	2	2	1	42	2
41	5	4	3	4	3	3	4	4	3	3	2	2	1	43	2
42	5	4	3	4	3	3	4	4	3	3	2	3	1	43	2
43	5	5	3	4	3	3	4	4	3	3	2	3	1	44	2
44	5	5	3	4	3	3	4	4	3	3	2	3	2	44	2
45	5	5	3	4	3	3	4	4	4	3	2	3	2	45	2
46	5	5	3	4	3	3	4	5	4	3	2	3	2	45	2
47	5	5	3	4	3	4	4	5	4	3	2	3	2	46	2
48	6	5	3	4	3	4	4	5	4	3	2	3	2	46	2
49	6	5	3	4	3	4	5	5	4	3	2	3	2	47	2
50	6	5	3	5	3	4	5	5	4	3	2	3	2	47	2

MOTOR ITEMS:

A EATING
B GROOMING
C BATHING
D DRESSING—UPPER BODY
E DRESSING—LOWER BODY
F TOILETING
G BLADDER—MANAGEMENT
H BOWEL MANAGEMENT
I TRANSFER-BED, CHAIR, WHEELCHAIR
J TRANSFER TOILET
K TRANSFER TUB/SHOWER
L WALK/WHEELCHAIR
M STAIRS

entering incorrect codes, and online help is available about the fields to be coded. This new tool allows the users to provide more accurate data to the UDSMR and helps to further standardize the tool for clinical and research use. FIMware allows for easy transfer of data to the UDSMR by disk, and also allows users at the clinical sites to compare their patient data with national outcome data to gauge patient progress.

Recent research has resulted in the use of the standardized FIM to categorize rehabilitation inpatients by their length of stay in medical rehabilitation [15]. This recent research has suggested that the FIM be used to replace the current system of Tax Equity and Fiscal Responsibility Act (TEFRA) reimbursement for services with a Function-Related Groups (FRGs) system, which would be more appropriate for medical rehabilitation services and patients. This development of an FRG system for medical rehabilitation has allowed the UDSMR to incorporate FRGs into the FIMware for reference by users in the field. Only through the use of consistent and standardized

Table 1. *Continued.*

FIM Score	A	B	C	D	E	F	G	H	I	J	K	L	M	0-100 Meas	S.E.
				MOTOR				ITEMS							
51	6	5	3	5	3	4	5	5	4	4	2	3	2	48	2
52	6	5	3	5	3	4	5	5	4	4	3	3	2	49	2
53	6	5	4	5	3	4	5	5	4	4	3	3	2	49	2
54	6	5	4	5	4	4	5	5	4	4	3	3	2	50	2
55	6	5	4	5	4	4	5	5	4	4	3	4	2	50	2
56	6	6	4	5	4	4	5	5	4	4	3	4	2	51	2
57	6	6	4	5	4	4	5	5	5	4	3	4	2	51	2
58	6	6	4	5	4	5	5	5	5	4	3	4	2	52	2
59	6	6	4	5	4	5	5	6	5	4	3	4	2	52	2
60	6	6	4	5	4	5	5	6	5	5	3	4	2	53	2
61	6	6	4	5	4	5	6	6	5	5	3	4	2	53	2
62	6	6	4	5	4	5	6	6	5	5	3	4	3	54	2
63	6	6	4	5	4	5	6	6	5	5	4	4	3	55	2
64	6	6	4	6	4	5	6	6	5	5	4	4	3	55	2
65	6	6	5	6	4	5	6	6	5	5	4	4	3	56	2
66	6	6	5	6	5	5	6	6	5	5	4	4	3	56	2
67	6	6	5	6	5	5	6	6	5	5	4	5	3	57	2
68	7	6	5	6	5	5	6	6	5	5	4	5	3	58	3
69	7	6	5	6	5	5	6	6	6	5	4	5	3	58	3
70	7	6	5	6	5	6	6	6	6	5	4	5	3	59	3
71	7	6	5	6	5	6	6	6	6	5	4	5	4	60	3
72	7	6	5	6	5	6	6	6	6	5	5	5	4	60	3
73	7	6	5	6	5	6	6	6	6	6	5	5	4	61	3
74	7	6	6	6	5	6	6	6	6	6	5	5	4	62	3
75	7	6	6	6	6	6	6	6	6	6	5	5	4	62	3
76	7	7	6	6	6	6	6	6	6	6	5	5	4	63	3
77	7	7	6	6	6	6	6	6	6	6	5	6	4	64	3
78	7	7	6	6	6	6	6	7	6	6	5	6	4	65	3
79	7	7	6	6	6	6	7	7	6	6	5	6	4	66	3
80	7	7	6	7	6	6	7	7	6	6	5	6	4	67	3
81	7	7	6	7	6	6	7	7	6	6	5	6	5	68	3
82	7	7	6	7	6	6	7	7	6	6	6	6	5	69	4
83	7	7	6	7	6	6	7	7	7	6	6	6	5	70	4
84	7	7	6	7	6	7	7	7	7	6	6	6	5	72	4
85	7	7	6	7	6	7	7	7	7	7	6	6	5	73	4
86	7	7	7	7	6	7	7	7	7	7	6	6	5	75	5
87	7	7	7	7	7	7	7	7	7	7	6	6	5	77	5
88	7	7	7	7	7	7	7	7	7	7	6	6	6	80	6
89	7	7	7	7	7	7	7	7	7	7	6	7	6	84	7
90	7	7	7	7	7	7	7	7	7	7	7	7	6	90	10
91	7	7	7	7	7	7	7	7	7	7	7	7	7	100	10

MOTOR ITEMS:

A EATING
B GROOMING
C BATHING
D DRESSING—UPPER BODY
E DRESSING—LOWER BODY
F TOILETING
G BLADDER MANAGEMENT
H BOWEL MANAGEMENT
I TRANSFER—BED, CHAIR, WHEELCHAIR
J TRANSFER TOILET
K TRANSFER TUB/SHOWER
L WALK/WHEELCHAIR
M STAIRS

procedures for collection and interpretation of research results from clean data can such systems be legitimately developed and implemented in the field.

In addition to standardizing the use of the FIM through guides, newsletters, and FIMware, the UDSMR also requires that subscribing facilities pass a rigorous test of credentialing of their clinicians who use the FIM to be certain that they are well trained in its use. Training is an important part of the UDSMR, as each subscribing facility receives extensive training on the use of the FIM before the test for credentialing. Only those facilities that pass the two-phase credentialing test provided by the UDSMR may have their data aggregated in regional and national reports on patients provided to subscribers on a quarterly basis. The credentialing test in Phase 1 requires that clinicians take a written exam on three standardized case studies. Clinicians may pass this first phase only if they score above 80% correct on the scoring of the FIM items. In the second phase, the UDSMR verifies the accuracy of the data

Table 1. *Continued.*

FIM Score	Cognitive			Items		0–100	
	N	O	P	Q	R	Meas	S.E.
5	1	1	1	1	1	0	12
6	2	1	1	1	1	12	12
7	2	2	1	1	1	20	8
8	2	2	2	1	1	25	7
9	2	2	2	1	2	28	6
10	2	2	2	2	2	31	6
11	3	2	2	2	2	34	5
12	3	3	2	2	2	36	5
13	3	3	3	2	2	38	5
14	4	3	3	2	2	40	4
15	4	4	3	2	2	41	4
16	4	4	3	2	3	43	4
17	4	4	3	3	3	44	4
18	4	4	4	3	3	46	4
19	5	4	4	3	3	47	4
20	5	5	4	3	3	49	4
21	5	5	4	3	4	50	4
22	5	5	4	4	4	52	4
23	5	5	5	4	4	53	4
24	6	5	5	4	4	55	4
25	6	6	5	4	4	57	4
26	6	6	5	4	5	58	5
27	6	6	5	5	5	60	5
28	6	6	6	5	5	62	5
29	6	6	6	5	6	65	5
30	6	6	6	6	6	67	6
31	7	6	6	6	6	70	6
32	7	7	6	6	6	74	7
33	7	7	7	6	6	79	9
34	7	7	7	6	7	88	12
35	7	7	7	7	7	100	12

COGNITIVE ITEMS

N   COMPREHENSION
O   EXPRESSION
P   SOCIAL INTERACTION
Q   PROBLEM SOLVING
R   MEMORY

reported to it by comparing facility data to regional and national data to determine whether the data reported are comparable. Thus, the UDSMR ensures that FIM data are both standardized and reliable in a variety of ways.

This process works well for facilities who are subscribers to the UDSMR. However, the use of the FIM without training and credentialing is not encouraged, as the use of data collected from this or any tool without a clear understanding of its applications is not recommended. This is one of the important reasons why Johnston et al. [1] advocated the use of measurement standards in medical rehabilitation.

Is the Scale Reliable?

Numerous research studies have been performed on the FIM to determine its reliability and validity. Hamilton et al. [16] recently showed that the FIM is highly reliable in its use even by facilities that failed the credentialing process of the UDSMR. However, the reliability of the six subscales and the total scale in the hands of trained clinicians assessing their own patients at their own facilities was consistently shown to be greater than .90. This outstanding reliability of the FIM strongly encourages its use by clinicians with the proper training. The results of other studies (e.g., [17]) have shown similar results with regard to trained and untrained raters. Interrater reliabilities for the FIM are more than .90, and test–retest reliability has been shown to be over .80.

The most recent test of *interrater agreement* was performed by having two or more pairs of clinicians assess each of 863 patients undergoing inpatient medical rehabilitation at 74 UDS subscribing hospitals. The results were total FIM intraclass correlation coefficient (ANOVA) .96, self-care .93, sphincter control .90, mobility .91, locomotion .89, communication .89, and social cognition .88; FIM kappa mean was .56 (range, .49–.63) [16]. It was concluded that the seven-level FIM demonstrated good interrater agreement among clinicians. Efforts to improve and refine testing of interrater reliability are ongoing. This is important because further research in functional assessment is addressing use of the FIM to predict clinical outcomes and resource need.

Precision of the FIM (that is, the ability of the FIM to detect meaningful change in level of function) has been observed to be high. For a sample of 309 traumatic brain-injured (TBI) patients admitted to five TBI Model Systems hospitals in the United States, the admission FIM average score was 59 with a 95% confidence range of ±3.2. Discharge FIM average score was 100 with a 95% confidence range of ±2.8 [18].

Feasibility of use of the FIM has been observed to be acceptable. Feasibility may be estimated by documenting the learning time and administration time for a clinician using the instrument. During the implementation phase the average time to learn to use the FIM was reported to be close to 60 min and the time to evaluate a patient was about 30 min. Telephone interviews used to assess function on the FIM take approximately 20–30 min.

In summary, studies to date indicate that the FIM has reliability, clinically appropriate validity, interrater agreement, precision, and feasibility.

Is the Scale Valid?

The validity of a scale may be assessed in a number of ways. The FIM has been shown to have face validity, as it was constructed by a multidisciplinary team in response to the task force. The FIM is unique in its implementation across so widespread a group of medical rehabilitation facilities at both the national and international levels. However, more rigorous psychometric tests of the validity of the FIM have examined its predictive validity.

Predictive validity is the extent to which a scale can predict outcomes that are related to the domain measured by the scale. Thus, for medical rehabilitation, the key outcomes of interest for the predictive validity of the FIM include both the burden of care for the patients and the ability of the FIM to predict discharge status, length of stay, and severity of disability.

Several studies have shown the FIM to be the best predictor of burden of care for multiple sclerosis stroke, and head-injured patients [19,20,21]. These studies revealed that the FIM outperformed several other common standardized, reliable, and valid instruments used in the field to measure patient severity in medical rehabilitation. When predicting the number of minutes of help per day required for such patient groups, the FIM total score and its subscales and items outperformed the Environmental Status Scale (ESS), Incapacity Status Scale (ISS), Sickness Impact Profile (SIP), and others.

The results of the Stineman et al. [15] study with regard to FRGs predicting categories of length of stay showed that FIM scores at admission in combination with patient age were the only factors necessary to outperform other models in determining length of stay categories in patients within impairment categories. Patient FIM scores at admission for motor and cognitive areas separately were the only factors predictive of length of stay within impairment categories when given the age of the patient.

Granger et al. [22] have shown that the FIM is also a key predictor of discharge status in stroke patients. The FIM varied directly with the percentage of patients discharged to the community; the higher the FIM score was at discharge from medical rehabilitation, the more likely the patient was to be discharged to the community. Fewer than half of the stroke patients discharged with FIM scores less than 60 returned to the community, while more than 90% of those with FIM scores greater than 100 returned to the community.

These studies clearly show that the FIM has predictive validity. However, predictive validity is only one of many types of validity, and the FIM has been shown to have content validity as well. The Rasch studies of the FIM have shown the scale to be composed of two unidimensional measures of cognitive and motor functioning. The Rasch analysis of a scale for its usefulness requires that the scale measure what it was intended to measure in only one dimension, that is, only one dimension at a time. The studies of the FIM by Granger et al. [12], Heinemann et al. [13,23], and Linacre et al. [14] showed that the scale has unidimensionality and thus content validity. The items in the motor area form a clear interval continuum in their difficulties, thus allowing individuals to be placed along the continuum based on their abilities to function independently in the motor domain. Likewise, the cognitive items form a second continuum that allows individuals to be placed along that interval-level continuum as well.

In summary, the FIM and its use within the UDSMR has provided a useful example of a scale that has received considerable attention with regard to its measurement properties. The FIM has been shown to be practical for clinical use, standardized, reliable, and valid, with high interrater reliability on individual items, subscales, domains, and total scores, and with powerful predictive validity across the key outcomes of medical rehabilitation. Further studies of existing scales need to follow this process to determine their usefulness in determining the outcomes of medical rehabilitation. To the extent that a scale can be shown to be reliable, and to predict the outcomes of interest in the field, the scale may be said to meet the measurement standards that determine its value. We are aware of limitations of the FIM in fully describing the characteristics of disability in patients recovering from head injury and those with high quadriplegia from spinal cord injury. There is need for some technical refinements with respect to assessment criteria for bladder, bowel, locomotion, comprehension, expression, and stair climbing.

The raw scores are not linear and should not be used in parametric statistical analyses [12]. There is current controversy involving the appropriate mathematical treatment of such scales when they are used to establish parameters for practice, quality assurance, and program evaluation. Merbitz et al. [2] are credited with precipitating a closer look at functional status scales that have ordinal rather than equal interval characteristics. They argued that data obtained from an ordinal scale would not allow mathematical operations which could directly relate to the real world, and they contended that results of mathematical manipulations performed on ordinal data were not logically valid and could be misinterpreted. Wright and Linacre [24] proposed a Rasch transformation of ordinal functional status scores into a linear ratio scale so that mathematical operations could be conducted. Harvey et al. [25] stressed that interval measurement would improve functional status scales by providing unidimensionality and additivity. Unidimensionality means that items progress in difficulty across a common range of performance, each item poses a constant level of difficulty for the subjects, and the abilities of subjects can be located according to a common standard. Additivity means that adding one more unit always increases the pool by the same amount.

Using a Rasch-transformed measure permits statistical validity in comparing individuals on the basis of results using an aggregate score of a scale and permits valid comparison of change in aggregate scores over time. Rasch analysis of the FIM has shown that it has motor and cognitive components that each have unidirectional characteristics, additivity, and good reliability. Rasch-converted measures are available. However, it remains to be empirically tested how importantly and to what degree this may affect results of research studies.

What is in the Future of the FIM?

With periodic reassessment, changes in patient performance over time can be measured and rehabilitation outcomes determined. There are many uses for this kind of information. With the advent of cost containment and the need for more efficient and effective programs, managers and administrators are looking to patient improvement as an indicator of institutional productivity. In the past, such information has not been available. Use of the FIM and the Uniform Data Set will provide medical rehabilitation with critical, timely information that has multiple purposes, including common language and definitions by which the industry can communicate and normative data that will permit assessment of effectiveness and cost efficiency of care. These have important implications for improving patient outcomes and management of care resources.

In addition, clinical and administrative feedback information is provided that can facilitate planning, evaluation, and policy decisions, and will satisfy requirements of accrediting bodies for quality assurance and program evaluation. Further, the research and education implications of uniform clinical data are substantial. Concurrently there is a practical, strong economic incentive because of the probable change in Medicare reimbursement from a cost basis to a prospective system, which means pre-price packaging. Presumably, facilities will be rewarded for precise goal-setting and efficiency in achieving their rehabilitation goals. It is possible that the UDSMR or some component will be a potent determinant of how a prospective payment system for medical rehabilitation may be shaped. This avenue of research is being explored by Stineman and co-workers, who have developed the FRG technology [15]. FRGs is a system for classifying patients in a way to predict length of stay and may be used to help in clinical and facility management as well as to form a basis for prospective payment.

References

1. Johnston MV, Keith RA, Hinderer SR (1992) Measurement standards for interdisciplinary medical rehabilitation. Arch Phys Med Rehabil 73:S3–S23

2. Merbitz C, Morris J, Grip JC (1989) Ordinal scales and foundations of misinference. Arch Phys Med Rehabil 70:308–312
3. Guide for the Uniform Data Set for Medical Rehabilitation (Adult FIM™) version 4.0. (1993) State University of New York at Buffalo, Buffalo, NY
4. Nagi SZ (1965) Disability and rehabilitation. Ohio State University Press, Columbus
5. World Health Organization (1980) International classification of impairments, disabilities, and handicaps: A manual of classification relating to the consequences of disease (ICIDH). World Health Organization, Geneva
6. Maslow AH (1954) Motivation and personality. Harper and Row, New York
7. von Bertalanffy L (1968) General system theory; foundations, development, applications. Braziller, New York
8. Kielhofner G, Burke JP (1980) A model of human occupation, Part 1. Conceptual framework and content. Am J Occup Ther 34:572–581
9. Granger CV, Hamilton BB (1992) UDS report: The Uniform Data System for Medical Rehabilitation report of first admissions for 1990. Am J Phys Med Rehabil 71:108–113
10. Granger CV, Hamilton BB (1993) The Uniform Data System for Medical Rehabilitation report of first admissions for 1991. Am J Phys Med Rehabil 72:33–38
11. Hamilton BB, Granger CV, Sherwin FS, Zielezny M, Tashman JS (1987) A uniform national data system for medical rehabilitation. In: Fuhrer MJ (ed) Rehabilitation outcomes: analysis and measurement. Brookes, Baltimore, pp 137–147
12. Granger CV, Hamilton BB, Linacre JM, Heinemann AW, Wright BD (1993) Performance profiles of the Functional Independence Measure. Am J Phys Med Rehabil 72:84–89
13. Heinemann AW, Hamilton BB, Granger CV, Linacre JM, Wright BD (1992) Rehabilitation efficacy for brain and spinal cord injury—final report. Project R49/CCR503609. Rehabilitation Institute of Chicago, Centers for Disease Control, Chicago
14. Linacre JM, Heinemann AW, Wright BD, Granger CV, Hamilton BB (1994) The structure and stability of the Functional Independence Measure. Arch Phys Med Rehabil 75:127–132
15. Stineman MG, Escarce JJ, Goin JE, Hamilton BB, Granger CV, Williams SV (1992) Function related groups (FRGs): a patient classification system for medical rehabilitation (abstract). Arch Phys Med Rehabil 73:957
16. Hamilton BB, Fiedler RC, Laughlin JA, Granger CV (1994) Interrater reliability of the 7-level functional independence measure (FIM). Scand J Rehab Med 26:115–119
17. Byrnes MB, Powers FF (1989) FIM: its use in identifying rehabilitation needs in the head-injured patient. J Neurosci Nurs 21(1):61–63
18. Dahmer ER, Shilling MA, Hamilton BB, Bontke CF, Englander J, Kreutzer JS, Ragnarsson KT, Rosenthal M (1993) A model systems database for traumatic brain injury. J Head Trauma Rehabil 8:12–25
19. Granger CV, Cotter AC, Hamilton BB, Fiedler RC, Hens MM (1990) Functional assessment scales: a study of persons with multiple sclerosis. Arch Phys Med Rehabil 71:870–875
20. Granger CV, Cotter AC, Hamilton BB, Fiedler RC (1993) Functional assessment scales: a study of persons after stroke. Arch Phys Med Rehabil 74:133–138
21. Granger CV, Divan N, Fiedler RC (1995) Functional assessment scales: a study of persons after traumatic brain injury. Am J Phys Med Rehabil 74:107–113
22. Granger CV, Hamilton BB, Fiedler RC (1992) Discharge outcome after stroke rehabilitation. Stroke 23:978–982
23. Heinemann AW, Linacre JM, Wright BD, Hamilton BB, Granger CV (1994) Measurement characteristics of the Functional Independence Measure (FIM). Top Stroke Rehabil 1:1–15
24. Wright BD, Linacre JM (1989) Observations are always ordinal; measurements, however, must be interval. Arch Phys Med Rehabil 70:857–860
25. Harvey RF, Silverstein B, Venzon MM, Kilgore KM, Fisher WP, Steiner M, Harley JP (1992) Applying psychometric criteria to functional assessment in medical rehabilitation: III. Construct validity and predicting level of care. Arch Phys Med Rehabil 73:887–892

Prognostication in Stroke Rehabilitation

Murray E. Brandstater

Summary. Good early prediction of ultimate outcome following stroke rehabilitation benefits patients and health care professionals. Numerous research studies have reported stroke outcomes, but the conclusions are not always in agreement because of differences in study methodology and in patient characteristics. However, some general conclusions about prognostication can be made. Early survival is poorer in those patients who have cerebral hemorrhage, coma at onset, or heart disease. Recovery from neurological impairment such as hemiplegia is influenced by lesion-related variables such as lesion size and location. Recovery from hemiplegia follows a predictable pattern, with most motor recovery occurring within the first 6 months. The disability status of stroke patients at late follow-up depends most on initial activities of daily living (ADL) scores recorded post onset. Characteristics that predict a less favorable outcome are older age and presence of urinary incontinence, bowel incontinence, and visuospatial deficits. Social and psychological variables, especially prestroke family interaction and presence of an able spouse, may strongly influence ultimate disability status and the return of patients to their home.

Introduction

Prognostication regarding outcome for a stroke patient is often expressed in the simple question—"Is this patient a good candidate for rehabilitation?" The benefits of good prognostication are self-evident. Patients and family members need to know the prospects for survival, the degree of recovery that may be expected, and the extent of possible residual disability following rehabilitation. Professionals providing care need information with which to counsel patients and families. Knowledge of prognosis of individual patients can guide physicians and therapists in selection of specific therapies and appropriate intensities of therapy. Finally, good prognostication can help to reduce costs of care through reduction of misdirected therapy and optimal use of facilities and staff.

Numerous studies over many years have reported outcomes of patients following stroke. Analysis of the information from those studies prompted attempts to define

[1]Department of Physical Medicine and Rehabilitation, Loma Linda University, 11234 Anderson Street, Loma Linda, CA 92354 USA

variables that would predict outcomes. However, accurate prognostication of the ultimate status of patients after recovery from stroke has proven to be elusive. The following issues represent some of the difficulties encountered in stroke outcome research: the effects of cerebrovascular disease are heterogeneous; pathologies differ; some patients have only transient symptoms, while in others the clinical manifestations occur abruptly and are accompanied by severe impairment. Many studies are not comparable; e.g., it is difficult to compare studies that aggregate all patients regardless of pathology, lesion site, time interval since onset, and degree of impairment with those studies of selected subgroups of patients.

A major limitation in interpretation of many early reports on prediction of stroke outcome has been poor definition of prognostic variables and outcome variables. Methodological issues in stroke outcome research were reviewed in a symposium in 1989 [1,2]. Important recommendations were made to standardize methodologies in outcome studies in stroke research [3], and in 1989 a World Health Organization (WHO) task force issued similar recommendations [4].

Prognostic Indicators

Many variables may influence the survival, recovery, and ultimate outcome of an individual who has sustained an acute stroke. These variables may be categorized into those that are patient related, those that are lesion related, those that are intervention- and therapy related, and those that are psychosocial. A classification of these variables is given in Table 1.

Patient Demographic Variables

Typical demographic variables that have been included in outcome studies of stroke are age, gender, and race.

Table 1. Classification of prognostic variables.

Patient demographic variables
General medical characteristics
   Examples: hypertension, heart disease, diabetes
Lesion-related variables
   Pathology
   Lesion site and size
   Impairment characteristics
   Coma at onset
   Bladder and bowel continence
Specific therapy interventions
   Nature of therapy
   Time of initiating therapy
   Intensity of therapy
Psychosocial variables
   Socioeconomic status
   Premorbid personality
   Patient family role

General Medical Characteristics

Numerous risk factors for stroke have been identified, namely, hypertension, diabetes, heart disease, atrial fibrillation, elevated blood lipids, obesity, past history of stroke, physical inactivity, estrogen therapy, high alcohol consumption, and history of smoking. Besides being a risk factor for stroke, heart disease influences early survival. All these risk factors increase the likelihood of recurrent stroke and hence will influence long-term survival.

Some medical conditions have a direct effect on functional recovery and ultimate functional status. Some disorders, such as congestive heart failure, limit the capacity of the patient to engage in all aspects of the rehabilitation program or to exercise at a sufficient level of intensity to realize maximum benefit. Other conditions may contribute additional impairments and compound the patient's disabilities, such as osteoarthritis of the hips and knees, arthropathy from rheumatoid arthritis, polyneuropathy, amputation, and gross obesity.

Lesion-Related Variables

The pathology of the stroke, hemorrhage versus infarction, has an important impact on short-term poststroke survival. Early survival also depends on the severity of the lesion, which is determined by its size and the extent of neurological deficits. The occurrence of coma at stroke onset reflects severity and is an important predictor of 30-day survival. Other characteristics of the lesion that influence the outcome are its location (cortex versus subcortex or brainstem) and the specific impairments (severity of paralysis, presence of visuospatial deficits, urinary incontinence, bowel incontinence).

Specific Therapy Interventions

The degree of patient recovery and functional outcome depend on a number of factors related to the rehabilitation program. Therapy interventions that influence outcome are whether a patient receives a rehabilitation program, time interval from stroke onset to beginning of therapy, and whether rehabilitation consists of a coordinated program of comprehensive therapy.

Psychosocial Variables

The socioeconomic status of the patient, the role of the individual within the family, the degree of family support, and the patient's premorbid personality are all factors that may influence outcome.

Outcome Variables

The outcome of patients who sustain a stroke may be defined within different domains. A list of some outcome variables is shown in Table 2. Each prognostic indicator has its own effect on these outcome variables. For example, stroke pathology affects early survival while rehabilitation therapy affects the ultimate degree of disability. The size or extent of the lesion may affect both survival and ultimate disability status.

Table 2. Outcome variables.

Survival
Impairment: neurological deficit
  Degree of paralysis
  Aphasia
  Visual field defect, neglect
Disability
  Activities of daily living (ADL)
  Ambulation
Social variables
  Discharge destination
  Living arrangements
  Social integration

Predicting Outcome

Survival

Early death following a stroke is usually related to the underlying pathology and to the severity of the lesion. The 30-day survival for patients with cerebral infarction is 85%, but for patients with intracerebral hemorrhage survival is reported to be 20%–52% [5,6]. Better management of cardiac and respiratory disorders has decreased mortality because of these associated diseases in the acute phase. Hypertension, heart disease, and diabetes however remain as risk factors for recurrence of stroke. Overall, the risk of recurrence of cerebral infarction in those patients who survive a stroke is about 6% of the patient population per year [7]. Coma following stroke onset is a poor prognostic sign, presumably because coma occurs frequently in cerebral hemorrhage, and also because a severe lesion with cerebral edema accompanies cerebral infarction.

Impairment

A wide range of neurological deficits is observed in acute stroke patients. The nature and severity of these deficits reflect the size and location of the underlying lesion. The initial severity of the neurological deficit is the most important determinant of residual impairment following recovery [8]. Recovery in impairment from stroke is based on neurological recovery. Adaptation by the patient, e.g., learning new techniques in self-care through training, may improve function but does not alter levels of impairment when a particular impairment is measured objectively.

Initial evaluation of impairments for purposes of predicting their recovery is best made between 1 and 3 weeks post onset. Observations made in the first several days may not be fully representative of lesion severity because deficits from minor lesions may be transient and resolve relatively quickly, while coma, confusion, or severe aphasia, when present, interfere with meaningful patient examination.

Hemiparesis and motor recovery are the most studied of all stroke impairments. As many as 88% of patients initially present with hemiparesis [9]. Motor recovery follows a fairly predictable pattern [10]. At onset, the arm is usually more involved than the leg, and eventual motor recovery in the arm is usually less than in the leg. Several authors have noted that the severity of arm weakness at onset, and the timing of return of movement, are both important predictors of eventual motor recovery in the arm [11–13]. The prognosis for return of useful hand function is poor when there is complete arm paralysis at onset or no measurable grip strength by 4 weeks [10,14]. However, even among those patients with severe arm weakness at onset, as many as 9% may gain good recovery of hand function. Most motor recovery occurs within the first 3 months [15,16], but when patients have partial return of voluntary movement continued progress may extend over a longer time [17]. Some other generalizations may be made. For patients showing some motor recovery in the hand by 4 weeks, as many as 70% will make a full or good recovery [11]. Full recovery, when it occurs, is usually complete within 3 months of onset. Bard and Hirshberg [11] claimed that "if no initial motion is noticed during the first 3 weeks, or if motion in one segment is not followed within a week by the appearance of motion in a second segment, the prognosis for recovery of full motion is poor."

The course of motor recovery reaches a plateau after an early phase of progressive improvement. Most recovery takes place in the first 3 months, and only minor additional measurable improvement occurs after 6 months post onset. By 6 months post onset, about 50% of patients still have hemiparesis. In long-term survivors, those with persisting hemiparesis still number about 50% [18].

About one-third of patients with acute stroke have clinical features of aphasia [9]. Language function in many of these patients improves, and at 6 months or more post stroke only 12%–18% have identifiable aphasia [19,20]. Skilbeck et al. [21] reported that patients with aphasia continued to show some late improvement in language function, even beyond 1 year after their stroke. Patients who initially would be classified as having Broca's aphasia have a variable outcome. In patients with large hemisphere lesions, Broca's aphasia persists with little recovery, while patients with smaller lesions often show early progressive improvement, changing to a milder form of aphasia with anomia and word-finding difficulty [22]. Patients with global aphasia tend to progress slowly, with recovery in comprehension often improving more than expressive ability. Communicative ability of patients who initially have global aphasia may show improvement over a longer period of time, up to a year or more [21,23] post onset. Those patients with global aphasia associated with large lesions may show only minor recovery. Recovery however may be quite good in those patients with smaller lesions [22]. Language recovery in Wernicke's aphasia is variable.

Almost half of patients with a right hemisphere stroke have a hemianopic field deficit [24]. In some of these patients the visual field deficit resolved slowly over time, and according to Hier et al. [25], the median time to recovery from hemianopia was 32 weeks. Visual neglect frequently accompanies visual field deficits, although it also occurs with intact visual fields. Visual neglect is very common in patients with right hemisphere stroke. In the majority of patients the neglect eventually clears [26].

Disability: Functional Status

The key outcomes from a rehabilitation perspective are those that describe the disability status of the patient. The central thrust of the rehabilitation program is to lessen ultimate disability; therefore, considerable attention has been directed at the identification of factors that will predict the late functional status of the patient, especially with respect to walking and activities of daily living (ADL).

Most patients admitted to an inpatient stroke rehabilitation program in the postacute phase have hemiparesis of sufficient severity that walking is impossible.

Some recovery of leg function almost always occurs, and improvement in mobility follows. By 3 months post onset, 54%–80% of patients are independent in walking [21,27,28]. In a retrospective study of 248 patients with stroke treated at a rehabilitation center, Feigenson et al. [29] reported that 85% of patients were ambulatory at discharge.

The degree of recovery in walking ability depends on motor recovery [30]. As measured on the Brunnstrom scale for stages of motor recovery, very few patients who remain in stage 2 (minimal voluntary movement) regain the ability to walk; however, most patients in stage 3 (active flexion and extension synergies through range of motion) do eventually walk. Data from the Framingham cohort reported by Gresham et al. [18] indicate that long-term survivors of stroke show good recovery of functional mobility, with 80% being independent in mobility.

Most patients with significant neurological impairment who survive a stroke are dependent in basic ADL, i.e., bathing, dressing, feeding, toileting, grooming, and transfers. The capacity of individuals to perform these activities is scored on disability rating scales such as the functional independence measure (FIM) [31,32]. Almost all patients show improved function in ADL as recovery occurs. Most improvement is noted in the first 6 months [8,33], although as many as 5% of patients show measurable improvement to 12 months post onset [34,35]. Other patients may show some functionally worthwhile improvement beyond 6 months that the disability scales usually fail to detect because of heir limited sensitivity at the upper end of the functional range [36].

The levels of functional independence eventually reached by stroke patients after recovery as reported by different authors are variable, presumably because of differences between study populations and differences in methods of treatment, follow-up, and data reporting. In most reports, between 47% and 76% survivors achieved partial or total independence in ADL [8,29,33,37].

Most authors who have attempted to determine which factors predict ultimate ADL functional outcome have used multivariate analysis. Of many independent variables tested, those reported to have the most influence on outcome are listed in Table 3. In some studies, not all these factors were shown statistically to predict outcome status.

In many studies the age of the patient is observed to influence functional ADL outcome [8,33,38–40], elderly patients doing less well. The effect of age may be at least partly from related factors such as more frequent coimpairments. If elderly patients are less functional premorbidly, this alone could explain poorer outcomes following a

Table 3. Factors predicting ADL outcome.

Age
Comorbidities
   Myocardial infarction
   Diabetes mellitus
Severity of stroke
   Degree of weakness
   Sitting balance
   Visuospatial deficits
   Mental changes
   Incontinence
   Initial ADL scores
Time interval: onset to rehabilitation

stroke. Furthermore, elderly patients often do not receive as intensive therapy as younger patients, and they may be discharged from the rehabilitation program sooner. In a study designed to examine age as an independent prognostic factor, Wade et al. [41] did not find a correlation between age and functional ADL outcome at 6 months.

Some authors have reported the negative influence of coexisting heart disease [33,42,43] and diabetes [43]. When present, these comorbidities would increase the likelihood of recurrent stroke and may limit the patient's full participation in an intensive program. In one of these studies [42], patients were evaluated very early, at 48 h postonset. These comorbidities affect survival, but it is not known to what degree their presence influences functional recovery from the stroke.

Numerous studies have reported that the severity of the stroke, i.e., lesion-related variables, definitely influence functional outcome. Stroke severity has been described in terms of degree of weakness [29,33,42,43], reduced sitting balance [8,38], visuospatial impairment [29,44], mental changes [8,29,42], and incontinence [38,40]. Intuitively it would seem reasonable to assume that patients with more severe neurological deficits would have worse functional outcomes, but this is not necessarily the case when isolated neurological impairments are considered. For example, analysis of predictive variables has failed to show that patients with sensory deficits have a poorer ultimate outcome [29,38].

The severity of the neurological deficit is reflected in the overall ADL score, and most authors have reported that the initial ADL score is a good predictor of ultimate ADL function [8,29,33,34,37,38,43,45]. Patients admitted for rehabilitation with lower ADL scores do not have as good a functional outcome as patients who initially had higher admission ADL scores. However the relationship between low admission ADL score and degree of improvement in rehabilitation is less certain [46]. Many patients with lower ADL admission scores may show good gains on the ADL scale but still have a lower functional level at outcome.

It is generally accepted that early initiation of therapy is desirable. It is believed that early rehabilitation minimizes secondary complications such as contractures and deconditioning and helps motivation. Some outcome studies report that early initiation of therapy favorably influences outcome [29,43]. It is uncertain how much scientific reliance can be placed on these reports because of the problem of confounding variables. For example, patients with less severe deficits are more likely to begin therapy sooner than patients with severe deficits, and the less severely involved patients will have better outcomes regardless of when therapy begins.

It is not known whether higher intensity therapy as an independent variable improves ultimate functional recovery, although some circumstantial evidence suggests that it does. Randomized control trials have shown that patients have a better outcome when treated in a specialized stroke rehabilitation unit [47,48]. One factor that might contribute to the superiority of the stroke rehabilitation unit is the more intensive therapy offered by such facilities.

Social Variables

Some stroke survivors continue to have severe disability and are unable to return home. Reports indicate that 10%–29% of patients require institutionalization because of their need for physical care [19,33,49,50]. Patients most likely to require institutional care are those with severe stroke who need maximum physical assistance in

ADL and who have bowel or bladder incontinence [29]. However, psychosocial variables, especially prestroke family interaction [51] and the presence of an able spouse [50], also influence whether patients return home.

The physical and psychological sequelae of stroke have a significant influence on the overall quality of life for survivors. Patients socialize less and engage in fewer community activities than strokefree individuals of comparable age [18]. Following recovery, deterioration in the quality of life compared with prestroke status, is caused by both physical and psychological variables such as depression [37].

In summary, patients whose initial postonset ADL scores are higher have a better ultimate functional outcome. Furthermore, older age, or the presence of urinary incontinence, bowel incontinence, or visuospatial deficits predict a less favorable functional outcome. These conclusions are based on studies of large groups of patients within which there is considerable individual variation. When a clinician is confronted with the challenge of evaluating an individual patient, guidelines for predicting functional outcome are useful but are not precise because multiple variables interact. A patient who might be judged as having a good prognosis for functional outcome might do poorly because of a negative psychosocial factor. The best estimate of prognosis can only be made after a thorough and comprehensive evaluation of the patient's medical, neurological, functional, and psychosocial status. The clinician at the bedside is in the best position to formulate a prognosis and provide an answer to the question, "Is this patient a good candidate for rehabilitation?"

References

1. Gresham GE (1990) Past achievements and new directions in stroke outcome research. Stroke 21(suppl II):II1–II2
2. Jongbloed L (1990) Problems of methodologic heterogeneity in studies predicting disability after stroke. Stroke 21(suppl II):II-32–II-34
3. Task Force Recommendations (1990) Symposium recommendations for methodology in stroke outcome research. Stroke 21(suppl II):II-68–II-73
4. World Health Organization (1989) Stroke 1989. Recommendations on stroke prevention, diagnosis, and therapy: report of the WHO Taskforce on Stroke and Other Cerebrovascular Disorders. Stroke 20:1407–1431
5. Broderick JP, Phillips SJ, Whisnant JP, O'Fallon WM, Bergstralh EJ (1989) Incidence rates of stroke in the eighties: the end of the decline in stroke. Stroke 20:577–582
6. Sacco RL, Wolf PA, Kammel WB, McNamara PM (1982) Survival and recurrence following stroke: the Framingham study. Stroke 13:290–295
7. Baker RN, Schwartz WS, Ramseyer JC (1968) Prognosis among survivors of ischemic stroke. Neurology 18:933–941
8. Wade DT, Langton Hewer R (1987) Functional abilities after stroke: measurement, natural history and prognosis. J Neurol Neurosurg Psychiatry 50:177–182
9. Foulkes MA, Wolf PA, Price TR, Mohr JP, Hier DB (1988) The stroke data bank: design, methods, and baseline characteristics. Stroke 19:547–554
10. Twitchell TE (1951) The restoration of motor function following hemiplegia in man. Brain 74:443–480
11. Bard G, Hirshberg CG (1965) Recovery of voluntary motion in upper extremity following hemiplegia. Arch Phys Med Rehabil 46:567–572
12. Gowland C (1987) Management of hemiplegic upper limb. In: Brandstater ME, Basmajian (eds) Stroke rehabilitation. Williams and Wilkins, Baltimore
13. Wade DT, Langton Hewer R, Wood VA, Skilbeck CE, Ismail HM (1983) The hemiplegic arm after stroke: measurement and recovery. J Neurol Neurosurg Psychiatry 46:521–524

14. Heller A, Wade DT, Wood VA, Sunderland A, Langton Hewer R, Ward E (1987) Arm function after stroke: measurement and recovery over the first three months. J Neurol Neurosurg Psychiatry 50:714–719
15. Kelly-Hayes M, Wolf PA, Kase CS, Gresham GE, Kannel WB, D'Agostino RB (1989) Time course of functional recovery after stroke: the Framingham study. J Neurol Rehabil 3:65–70
16. Smith DL, Akhtar AJ, Garraway WM (1985) Motor function after stroke. Age Ageing 14:46–48
17. Ferrucci L, Bandinelli S, Guralnik JM, Lamponi M, Bertini C, Falchini M, Baroni A (1993) Recovery of functional status after stroke: a post-rehabilitation follow-up study. Stroke 24:200–205
18. Gresham GE, Fitzpatrick TE, Wolf PA, McNamara PM, Kannel WB, Dawber TR (1975) Residual disability in survivors of stroke: the Framingham study. N Engl J Med 293:954–956
19. Gresham GE, Phillips TF, Wolf PA, McNamara PM, Kannel WB, Dawber TR (1979) Epidemiologic profile of long-term stroke disability: the Framingham study. Arch Phys Med Rehabil 60:487–491
20. Wade DT, Langton Hewer R, David RM, Enderby PM (1986) Aphasia after stroke: natural history and associated deficits. J Neurol Neurosurg Psychiatry 49:11–16
21. Skilbeck CE, Wade DT, Hewer RL, Wood VA (1983) Recovery after stroke. J Neurol Neurosurg Psychiatry 46:5–8
22. Kertesz A (1987) Communication disorders. In: Brandstater ME, Basmajian JV (eds) Stroke rehabilitation. Williams and Wilkins, Baltimore
23. Sarno MT, Levita E (1979) Recovery in treated aphasia in the first year post-stroke. Stroke 10:663–670
24. Hier DB, Mondlock J, Caplan LR (1983) Behavioral abnormalities after right hemisphere stroke. Neurology 33:337–344
25. Hier DB, Mondlock J, Caplan LR (1983) Recovery of behavioral abnormalities after right hemisphere stroke. Neurology 33:345–350
26. Meerwaldt JD (1983) Spatial disorientation in right hemisphere infarction: a study of the speed of recovery. J Neurol Neurosurg Psychiatry 46:426–429
27. Chin PL, Rosie A, Irving M, Smith R (1982) Studies in hemiplegic gait. In: Rose FC (ed) Advances in stroke therapy. Raven Press, New York
28. Wade DT, Wood VA, Langton Hewer R (1985) Recovery after stroke—the first 3 months. J Neurol Neurosurg Psychiatry 48:7–13
29. Feigenson JS, McDowell FH, Meese P, McCarthy ML, Greenberg SD (1977) Factors influencing outcome and length of stay in a stroke rehabilitation unit. Stroke 8:651–656
30. Brandstater ME, deBruin H, Gowland C, Clarke B (1983) An analysis of temporal variables in hemiplegic gait. Arch Phys Med Rehabil 64:583–587
31. Keith RA, Granger CV, Hamilton BB, Sherwin FS (1987) The functional independence measure: a new tool for rehabilitation. In: Eisenberg MG, Grzesiak RC (eds) Advances in clinical rehabilitation, vol 1. Springer-Verlag, New York, pp 6–18
32. Guide for the Uniform Data Set for medical rehabilitation (Adult FIM, Version 4.0) (1993) State University of New York, Buffalo
33. Dombovy ML, Basford JR, Whisnant JP, Bergstralh EJ (1987) Disability and use of rehabilitation services follwoing stroke in Rochester, Minnesota 1975–1979. Stroke 18:830–836
34. Carroll D (1962) The disability in hemiplegia caused by cerebrovascular disease: serial study of 98 cases. J Chronic Dis 15:179–188
35. Andrews K, Brocklehurst JC, Richards B, Laycock PJ (1981) The rate of recovery from stroke and its measurement. Int Rehabil Med 3:155–161
36. Wade DT, Langton Hewer R, Skilbeck CE, David RM (1985) Stroke: a critical approach to diagnosis, treatment, and management. Year Book, Chicago, p 241
37. Ahlsiö B, Britton M, Murray V, Theorell T (1984) Disablement and quality of life after stroke. Stroke 15:886–890
38. Wade DT, Skilbeck CE, Langton Hewer R (1983) Predicting Barthel ADL score at 6 months after an acute stroke. Arch Phys Med Rehabil 64:24–28

39. Lehmann JF, DeLateur BJ, Fowler RS, Warren CG, Arnhold R, Schertzer G, Hurta R, Whitmore JJ, Masock AJ, Chambers KH (1975) Stroke rehabilitation: outcome and prediction. Arch Phys Med Rehabil 56:383–389

40. Jiminez J, Morgan PP (1979) Predicting improvement in stroke patients referred for inpatient rehabilitation. Can Med Assoc J 121:1481–1484

41. Wade DT, Langton Hewer R, Wood VA (1984) Stroke: the influence of age on outcome. Age Ageing 13:357–362

42. Fullerton KJ, MacKenzie G, Stout RW (1988) Prognostic indices in stroke. Q J Med 66:147–162

43. Shah S, Vanclay F, Cooper B (1989) Predicting discharge status at commencement of stroke rehabilitation. Stroke 20:766–769

44. Wade DT, Langton Hewer R, Wood VA (1984) Stroke: influence of patient's sex and side of weakness on outcome. Arch Phys Med Rehabil 65:513–516

45. Granger CV, Greer DS, Liset E, Coulowbe J, O'Brien E (1975) Measurement of outcomes of care for stroke patients. Stroke 6:34–41

46. Jongbloed L (1986) Prediction of function after stroke: a critical review. Stroke 17:765–776

47. Stevens RS, Ambler NR, Warren MD (1984) A randomized controlled trial of a stroke rehabilitation ward. Age Ageing 13:65–75

48. Sivenius J, Pyorala K, Heinonen OP, Salonen JT, Riekkinen P (1985) The significance of intensity of rehabilitation of stroke—a controlled trial. Stroke 16:928–931

49. Lehmann JF, DeLateur BJ, Fowler RS, Warren CG, Arnhold R, Schertzer G, Hurta R, Whittmore JJ, Massock AJ, Chambers KH (1975) Stroke: does rehabilitation affect outcome. Arch Phys Med Rehabil 56:375–382

50. Kelly-Hayes M, Wolf PA, Kannel WB, Sytkowski P, D'Agostino RB, Gresham GE (1988) Factors influencing survival and the need for institutionalization following stroke: the Framingham study. Arch Phys Med Rehabil 69:415–418

51. Evans RL, Bishop DS, Matlock AL, Stranahan S, Halar EM, Noonan WC (1987) Prestroke family interaction as a predictor of stroke outcome. Arch Phys Med Rehabil 68:508–512

Prognostication of Stroke Patients Using the Stroke Impairment Assessment Set and the Functional Independence Measure

Shigeru Sonoda, Eiichi Saitoh, Kazuhisa Domen, and Naoichi Chino[1]

Summary. Outcome prediction is one of the main issues in stroke rehabilitation. Although many predictors have been tested and a considerable number of statistical methods employed, none to date has resulted in a satisfactory method for prognosis. We have successfully predicted stroke outcome using regression analysis with the Stroke Impairment Assessment Set (SIAS), which we have developed, and the Functional Independence Measure (FIM). Our subjects were 192 stroke patients who had completed rehabilitation whose average number of days from stroke onset was 53.0; their mean length of hospital stay was 94.9 days. Subjects were divided into two groups according to the total FIM score on admission: less than 80 compared to 80 or more. Patterns of correlation coefficients between admission parameters and the discharge FIM score differed between the two groups. Regression equations were separately made in each group with independent variables of the SIAS, the FIM, and several other parameters (piecewise regression analysis). Adding the impairment scale, the SIAS, and related items to the disability scale as independent variables enhanced the correlation coefficient of piecewise regression from .85 to .93. Stroke outcome can be successfully predicted using piecewise regression with the SIAS and the FIM. Stratification of stroke patients by their admission FIM scores is effective for making a good prognosis. The SIAS proved to be an adequate set to score impairment.

Introduction

Numerous articles concerning stroke outcome prediction have been published [1–4]. Although many predictors have been used and a considerable number of statistical methods employed, a satisfactory method for prognosis of stroke patients has not yet been found [5–7].

Recent studies are inclined to predict final disabilities based on initial disabilities. For example, Wade predicted a Barthel score [8] at 6 months from onset using initial age, hemianopsia, urinary incontinence, motor deficit, and sitting balance. The combined correlation coefficient, however, reached only about .6 [1]. Heinemann summarized that variance predicted in previous reports ranged from .46 to .73 for functional

[1]Department of Rehabilitation Medicine, Keio University School of Medicine, 35 Shinanamachi, Shinjuku-ku, Tokyo 160, Japan

status at discharge, and his own multiple regression study using the Functional Independence Measure (FIM) [9,10] resulted in an adjusted variance of .6 for the motor subscale of the FIM and .67 for the cognitive subscale [2]. In these studies, disability was employed as an independent variable in preference to impairment, and prediction results were not as practical. Although disability may be a good predictor, is there no room for impairment as a predictor? Because disability is based on impairment, impairment must potentially include information other than disability.

Why did preceding studies fail to prove the importance of the impairment scale in making prognosis? The first reason is that the impairment scale used was insufficient. Degree of motor impairment has been measured by the Motricity Index [11], Brunnstrom stage [12], or intrainstitutional scales. The Motricity Index does not take into account the synergy pattern, and although Brunnstrom stage considers synergy, its lower extremity scale is multitask assessed and is inconvenient for detecting fine changes. As a comprehensive set for impairment, the Fugl–Meyer scale [13], the Chedoke–McMaster Stroke Assessment [14], the Canadian Neurological Scale [15], and the National Institutes of Health (NIH) stroke scale [15] have been developed. Because none contains effective measures of unaffected side function or of higher cortical function, and as the latter two apply rather rough scales to acute stage stroke patients, their effectiveness as predictors is limited.

For these conditions, we have developed the Stroke Impairment Assessment Set (SIAS), which contains 22 items: motor, tone, sensory, range of motion, pain, trunk, visuospatial, speech, and unaffected side [17]; its reliability and validity have been established [18,19]. The first aim of this chapter is to reconfirm the importance of impairment in predicting stroke outcomes using the SIAS and FIM.

As a second reason for failure to make good predictions, the heterogeneity of stroke patients [7] should be considered. Although preceding studies treated stroke patients as one group [1,2], predictors of functional outcome differ according to initial severity of the stroke [7]. In our view, the higher the activities of daily living (ADL) level of the patient, the more the motor impairment contributes to functional outcomes.

To examine this hypothesis, simple (ungrouped) regression analysis is first employed to find the cutoff point of the patients; piecewise (grouped) analysis is then performed (see following section). Methods and results are combined to demonstrate these processes of analysis in order.

Subjects

Subjects were 192 stroke patients who were admitted to Keio University and its affiliated hospitals in 1993 within 4 months from onset (Table 1). Patients who could not complete rehabilitation because of social situations or were transferred to acute care hospitals were eliminated. There were 113 male and 79 female patients with an average age on admission of 62.0 years old (SD, 11.9). There were 114 with cerebral infarction, 69 with cerebral bleeding, and 9 with subarachnoid hemorrhage; 95 patients had a right-side brain lesion. Average number of days from stroke onset was 53.0, and mean length of hospital stay was 94.9 days.

Patients were divided into two groups: group L (lower group) includes the patients whose total FIM score on admission was less than 80; other patients were classified as

Table 1. Subjects.

	All patients	Group L[a]	Group H[b]
Cases	192	62	130
Sex			
Male	113	37	76
Female	79	25	54
Age			
Average	61.97	64.16	60.93
SD	11.89	10.94	12.22
Minimal	14	37	14
Maximal	92	92	85
Disease			
Cerebral infarction	114	31	83
Cerebral bleeding	69	28	41
Subarachnoid hemorrhage	9	3	6
Affected side of brain			
Right	95	30	65
Left	97	32	65
Days from stroke onset			
Average	52.96	48.69	55.01
SD	31.31	34.25	29.71
Median	55	41.5	57
Minimal	1	2	1
Maximal	119	117	119
Length of stay			
Average	94.87	118.98	83.37
SD	52.39	57.17	45.88
Median	88	119	84

[a] Group L included patients whose total Functional Independence Measure (FIM) score at admission was less than 80.

[b] Group H included patients whose total FIM score at admission was 80 or more.

group H (higher group) (see Table 1). The cut-off point of 80 was derived from the results of a simple regression analysis that is described later.

Methods and Results

The SIAS and the FIM were measured in each patient at admission and on discharge.

The SIAS covers a wide spectrum of impairment, and its rating scales are zero to five (0–5) (in motor items) or zero to three (Table 2). Another chapter in this volume describes more details of its definition [17]. Subscales of the SIAS were employed for further statistical analysis. Motor function was divided into upper extremity motor (sum of two items) and lower extremity motor (sum of three items); pain was integrated into the sensory functions. Therefore, eight subscales, that is, upper extremity motor, lower extremity motor, tone, sensory, range of motion, trunk, higher cortical, and sound (unaffected) side, were used.

The FIM, which is the disability scale utilized by the Uniform Data System for Medical Rehabilitation (UDSMR) [10], was employed to measure disability. As shown in Table 3, the subscales of the FIM—self-care, sphincter control, transfers, locomo-

Table 2. Stroke Impairment Assessment Set (SIAS).

	Upper extremity	Lower extremity
Motor		
Proximal	0–5	0–5 (hip)
		0–5 (knee)
Distal	0–5	0–5
Muscle tone		
DTRs	0–3	0–3
Muscle tone	0–3	0–3
Sensory		
Light touch	0–3	0–3
Position	0–3	0–3
Range of motion	0–3	0–3
Pain	0–3	
Trunk		
Verticality	0–3	
Abdominal	0–3	
Higher cortical		
Visuospatial	0–3	
Speech	0–3	
Unaffected side	0–3	0–3
Total	76	

DTR, Deep tendon reflex.

tion, communication, and social cognition—were used for further statistical consideration.

In addition, age and days from stroke onset were evaluated at admission because these factors were demonstrated to be important in a preliminary study. Understanding of the importance of attending gym sessions at admission was measured by a three-point scale. Those patients participating in exercise without hesitation were rated as 2; those failing to proceed to the gym were scored as 0, and the remaining patients, whose behavior fell between these extremes, were rated as 1.

Major complications/comorbidities (COMPLI) such as shoulder-hand syndrome, dementia, sufficient osteoarthritis to cause gait difficulty, or liver dysfunction so severe as to restrict the patient to bed were also rated. Patients with COMPLI were divided into three classes. Patients having no COMPLI that influenced the outcome of their stroke were assigned 0; those with COMPLI throughout the hospital stay were scored as 1. Any COMPLI that was tentative and only lowered the admission data was scored as −1; examples are an initial state of confusion or a shoulder-hand syndrome with associated pain that usually disappeared by discharge.

All statistical analyses as described here were performed by Statistica™ (Statsoft, Tulsa, OK, USA). Missing data were substituted by using the mean values of all patients.

Structure of the SIAS

Factor analysis included using all items of the SIAS on admission. Factors were rotated to a varimax solution. Coefficient values in each factor were connected as a line graph.

Table 3. Functional Independence Measure (FIM).

FIM Motor Items
  Self-care
    Eating
    Grooming
    Bathing
    Dressing, upper body
    Dressing, lower body
    Toileting
  Sphincter Control
    Bladder management
    Bowel management
  Transfers
    Bed, chair, wheelchair transfer
    Toilet transfer
    Tub, shower transfer
  Locomotion
    Walk/wheelchair
    Stairs
FIM Cognitive Items
  Communication
    Comprehension
    Expression
  Social cognition
    Social interaction
    Problem solving
    Memory
Scoring Criteria
  7: Complete independence
  6: Modified independence
  5: Supervision, setup
  4: Minimal assistance
  3: Moderate assistance
  2: Maximal assistance
  1: Total assistance

Factor analysis produced six factors with eugenvalues greater than 1. Figure 1 demonstrates these six factors as six lines. Note that each line has a high-value group of the items. Line 1 highlights the tone subscale and line 2 denotes high coefficients at trunk and unaffected side subscale. Similarly, five motor items, four sensory items, two range-of-motion items, and two higher cortical items comprise one group each. Thus, the subscales of the SIAS seem to be unidimensional.

Outcome Prediction (Simple Regression)

As a first step in looking for a good prediction method, the total FIM score at discharge was predicted using stepwise regression analysis. The admission FIM subscales and the SIAS subscales, age, and the days from onset were used as independent (explanatory) variables.

The predicted total FIM scores and the observed scores are plotted in Fig. 2a. The regression coefficient (r) was .80 and the adjusted r^2 was .62. The regression equation is not so fitted, as is depicted in the chart.

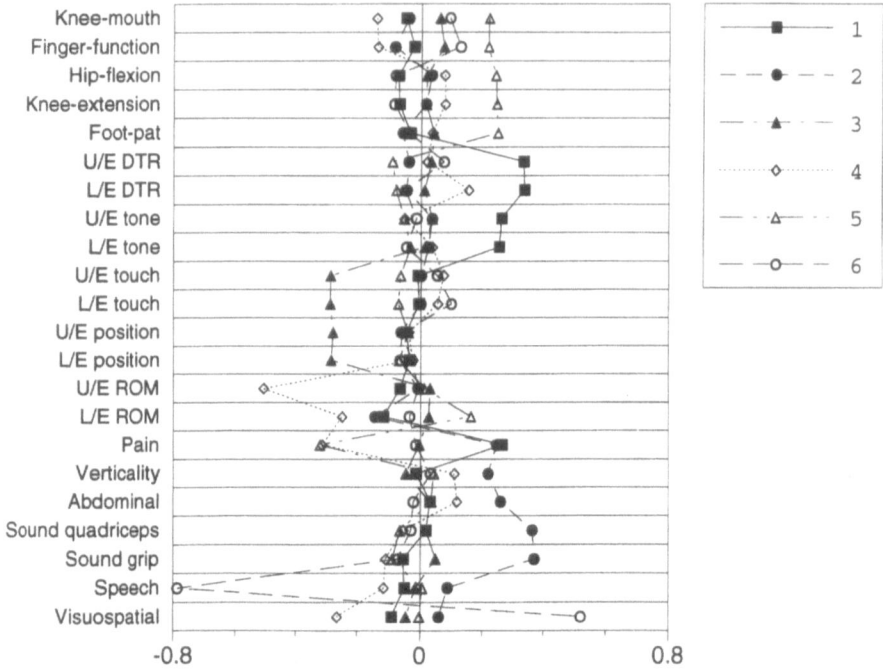

Fig. 1. Factor analysis of the Stroke Impairment Assessment Set (SIAS). The six lines denote each factor score coefficient from factor 1 to factor 6, obtained by factor analysis of the SIAS. Note each line's peak pattern of coefficients. *U/E*, upper extremity; *LE*, lower extremity; *DTR*, deep tendon reflex; *ROM*, range of motion

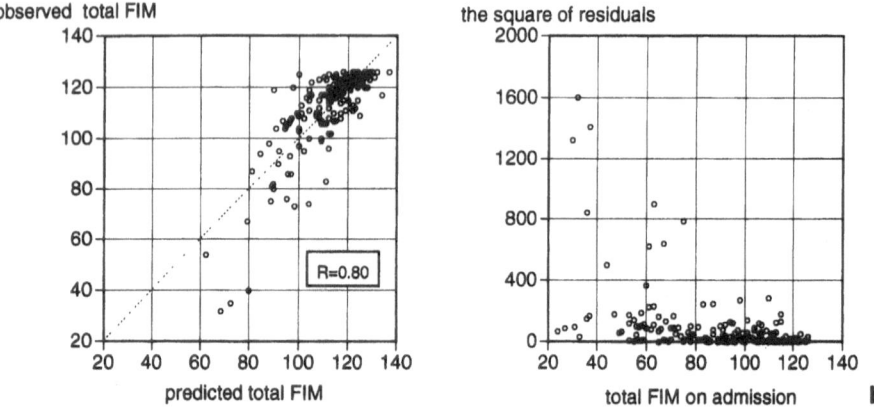

Fig. 2a,b. Simple regression analysis predicting the total Functional Independence Measure (FIM) at discharge. a Scattergram of predicted total FIM and observed total FIM at discharge. Each open circle indicates one patient. Regression coefficient was .80. b Residuals of simple regression analysis. Horizontal axis shows admission data, not discharge data. Note that all open circles more than 80 in total FIM score show small deviation

Next, residuals of the total FIM score at discharge were calculated to determine the cause of discrepancy. Figure 2b demonstrates the relationship between the square of the residuals and the admission total FIM scores. The residuals tended to be larger in patients whose total FIM score at admission was less than 80 (these patients comprise group L); group H, the group with higher FIM scores at admission, fit the regression equation relatively well.

Stratification of the Patients

To determine the characteristics of group L and group H, the contribution of the admission parameters to discharge outcomes was calculated using Spearman's rank correlation coefficients between FIM subtotal scores (motor and cognitive) at discharge and subscales (of the FIM or the SIAS) on admission, calculated in the two groups separately.

Figure 3a shows the correlation to the FIM motor subtotal score. In group L (open squares in the figure), the SIAS and the FIM had relatively low correlation to discharge FIM except to the cognitive subscores of the FIM. Group H (closed circles in the figure) revealed higher correlation at motor subscales of the SIAS and the FIM. In other words, motor impairment or motor disability has a strong effect on final (discharge) motor ability only in the group with higher ADL scores at admission. Thus the contribution of parameters on admission to the FIM motor subscale at discharge is affected by the admission FIM score.

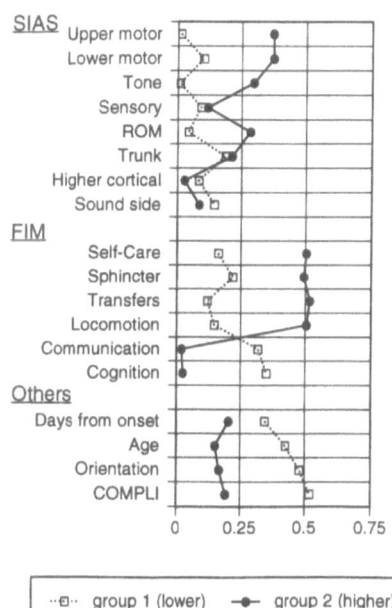
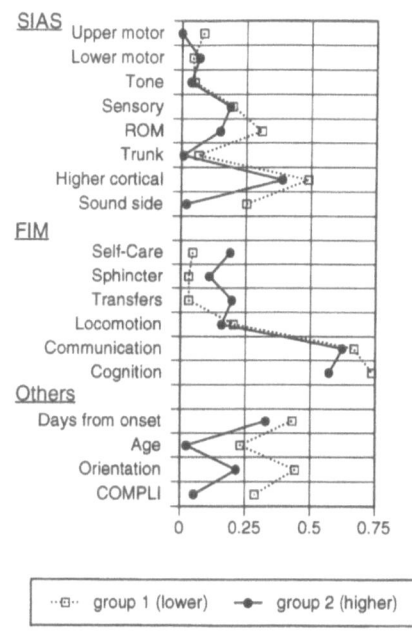

Fig. 3a,b. Spearman's rank correlation coefficient between FIM subtotal score at discharge and subscale score on admission. a Spearman's coefficient between FIM *motor* subtotal at discharge and subscales on admission. b Spearman's coefficient between FIM *cognitive* subtotal at discharge and subscales on admission. *COMPLI*, complication/comorbidity

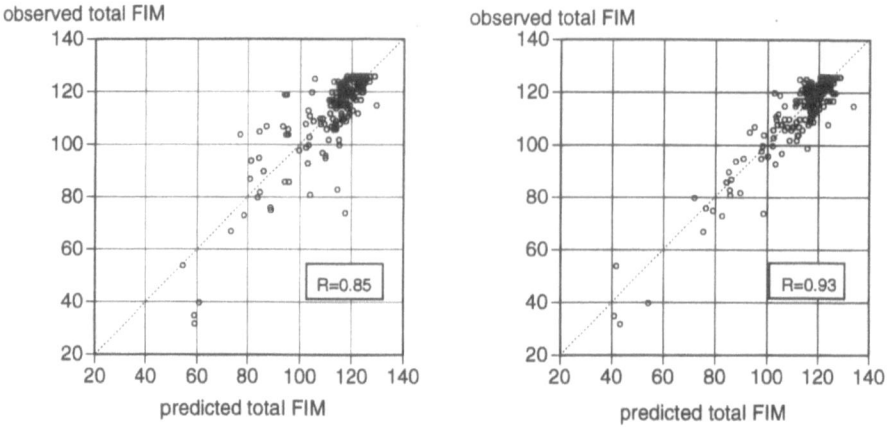

Fig. 4a,b. Piecewise regression analysis predicting the total FIM at discharge. Two regression equations were made according to the patients' total FIM score on admission. a As independent variables, FIM, age, and days from onset to admission are included; the SIAS, orientation, or complication are excluded. Correlation coefficient, .85. b Independent variables are SIAS, orientation, and complication, in addition to FIM, age, and days from onset to admission. Correlation coefficient increases to .93

On the other hand, both groups had similar patterns of correlation to the discharge cognitive FIM (Fig. 3b).

Outcome Prediction (Piecewise Regression)

To know whether adding impairment items to disability items as predictors increases the precision of the outcome prediction, stepwise regression analysis predicting the discharge total FIM score was carried out again with two sets of independent variables. The first set was composed of the subscores of FIM, age, and the days from stroke onset to admission; this set is referred to as the ADL set. The second set was made up of subscores of the SIAS, orientation to going to gym, and complications in addition to the first set, and is referred to as the full set.

Because a difference between the two groups was noticed, as has been described, two regression equations were combined in each variable set. The first regression equation is for group L patients and the second for group H patients.

Figure 4a shows the prediction results of the ADL set and Fig. 4b demonstrates the results of the full set. Results indicate that full set predicts better than the ADL set. The correlation coefficient is improved from .85 to .93 by adding the SIAS and other parameters to the ADL set variables. Table 4 shows the standardized partial regression coefficient for the full set.

Discussion

There are several points to be considered in successfully making the prognosis of stroke patients. The first consideration is the statistical methods employed. Second, the scales or items used should be suitable. The final point to be discussed is the timing of measurement of initial and final data.

Table 4. Piecewise regression parameters.

Dependent variables	B[a]	Beta[b]	P
Group L			
Age	−0.954	−0.48	.000
Communication	2.088	0.35	.000
COMPLI[c]	−10.943	−0.33	.000
Orientation	−11.728	−0.28	.001
Days from onset	−0.152	−0.24	.003
Sound side	−3.554	−0.21	.012
Trunk	2.494	0.19	.032
Tone	1.235	0.16	.037
Sensory	−0.846	−0.16	.035
Self-care	0.315	0.07	.305
Locomotion	1.270	0.07	.282
Higher cortical	1.556	0.07	.255
Group H			
Self-care	0.384	0.30	.002
Age	−0.164	−0.29	.000
Cognition	0.629	0.22	.011
Orientation	−11.714	−0.21	.001
Sphincter	0.890	0.21	.002
Days from onset	−0.048	−0.20	.003
Communication	0.654	0.20	.021
COMPLI[c]	−3.661	−0.20	.001
Ambulation	0.279	0.17	.049
Lower motor	0.327	0.16	.065
Transfer	−0.227	−0.11	.278
ROM	−0.531	−0.10	.130
Upper motor	0.216	0.09	.313

[a] Raw partial regression coefficient.
[b] Standardized partial regression coefficient.
[c] Complication/comorbidity.

Statistical Methods

Methods for outcome prediction have been changed in stroke rehabilitation. At first, simple correlation methods were employed and continence was recognized as a good predictor [5,6]. Because the existence of continence relates to the extent of the brain lesion, it certainly shows a fair basis on which to make prognosis, but this may not reach a practical level. Also, other significant predictors cannot be used alone [6].

Thereafter, regression analysis was frequently used, but in many cases with poor results [1–3,20]. Two factors can make prediction imprecise: the use of regression analysis itself and the variables used in the regression equation. The latter is discussed here later. Simple regression analysis may be inadequate because of the nonlinear nature of parameters in stroke patients.

There are two ways to avoid the disadvantage of regression analysis. One way is to discard it and to introduce newer methods, for example, decision theory [21] or the use of interval-scaled variables transferred by Rasch analysis [22,23]. These methods are promising. Further study, however, is needed before reaching conclusions as to the effectiveness of these methods because their precision is not yet very great [2,21].

Another way to improve precision is to stratify patients. Our study demonstrated that admission motor impairment contributes to the final outcome only in patients with high ADL at admission. Age and orientation are the key to improving disability for patients with lower ADL scores. These findings fit the clinical observations. The differences between high and low ADL groups at admission are large, so stratification seems to be critical. The change of correlation coefficient from .80 to .93 (from .64 to .86 by variance) demonstrates the importance of stratification.

Items

In this study, functional outcome is measured by the FIM at discharge. Because it is reasonable that the FIM at admission highly contributes to the final outcome, selection of items other than the FIM are discussed next.

The SIAS, which we have developed since 1990, was published in preliminary form in 1993 [17]. The SIAS can be completed by a single examiner requires only about 10 min to score all items. The weighted kappa value of the SIAS, which indicates interrater reliability, ranges from .30 to .98 [18,19]. Because the relatively low agreement appeared in the pain or verticality items in which most patients have a score of three, the lower kappa value seems to result from the algorithm of the kappa calculation [24]. Thus, the SIAS has fair to good interrater agreement and is also validated by several studies [17-19]. For example, motor items of the SIAS can detect finer changes than the Brunnstrom stage. The tape bisection visuospatial test item of the SIAS correlates to the line bisection test [19]. Also, the abdominal item, which can be measured in a sitting position, has a high correlation to the Daniels manual muscle testing (MMT) [19].

The piecewise regression result of this study demonstrated that adding the impairment scale and related items to the disability scale as independent variables enhanced the correlation coefficient from .85 to .93; that is, the precision of the outcome prediction improved. Some prediction studies using the impairment scales have showed lower precision than this study [1,25]. These studies used rather rough scales, that is, a narrower impairment measurement set than the SIAS. In other words, the SIAS can detect the proper part of the impairment that is not captured in the disability.

Measurement Timing

This study was conducted in Japan. Mean Japanese rehabilitation hospital admission is about 50 days from stroke onset and the length of stay is about 90 days, so that discharge status about 5 months from onset approximately denotes the final outcome. On the other hand, in the United States in 1992 the mean number of days from stroke onset to admission was 20 days and the mean length of stay in the rehabilitation hospital was 28 days, according to a report of the Uniform Data System for Medical Rehabilitation [26]. Although outcome studies performed in the Unites States frequently use the discharge status as the final outcome [2,4], the discharge status does not reveal the plateau level [7]. Thus, the timing of discharge in Japan is a critical advantage for prediction research.

Conclusion

Stroke outcome is successfully predicted using piecewise regression analysis with the SIAS, the FIM, patient orientation, and existence of complications. The correlation coefficient attained was .93. In outcome prediction, measuring both impairment and disability is important. Thus the SIAS has proved to be an adequate set to score impairment.

References

1. Wade DT, Skilbeck CE, Langton Hewer R (1983) Predicting Barthel ADL score at 6 months after an acute stroke. Arch Phys Med Rehabil 64:24–28
2. Heinemann AW, Linacre JM, Wright BD, Hamilton BB, Granger CV (1994) Prediction of rehabilitation outcomes with disability measures. Arch Phys Med Rehabil 75:133–143
3. Loewen SC, Anderson BA (1990) Predictors of stroke outcome using objective measurement scales. Stroke 21:78–81
4. Alexander MP (1994) Stroke rehabilitation outcome: a potential use of predictive variables to establish levels of care. Stroke 25:128–134
5. Wade DT (1992) Stroke: rehabilitation and long-term care. Lancet 339:791–793
6. Jongbloed L (1986) Prediction of function after stroke: a critical review. Stroke 17:765–776
7. Jongbloed L (1990) Problems of methodological heterogeneity in studies predicting disability after stroke. Stroke 21(Suppl II):II32–II34
8. Mahoney FI, Barthel DW (1965) Functional evaluation: the Barthel index. Md state Med J 14:61–65
9. Granger CV, Hamilition BB, Keith RA, Zielezny M, Sherwin FS (1986) Advances in functional assessment for medical rehabilitation. Top Geriatr Rehabil 1:59–74
10. Data management service of the Uniform Data System for Medical Rehabilitation and the Center for Functional Assessment Research (1990) Guide for use of the Uniform Data Set for Medical Rehabilitation, Version 3.1. State University of New York at Buffalo, Buffalo
11. Demeurisse G, Robaye E (1980) Motor evaluation in vascular hemiplegia. Eur Neurol 19:382–389
12. Brunnstrom S (1970) Movement therapy in hemiplegia: a neurophysiological approach. Harper and Row, New York
13. Fugl-Meyer AR, Jääskö L, Leyman I, Olsson S, Steglind S (1975) The post-stroke hemiplegic patient. I. a method for evaluation of physical performance. Scand J Rehabil Med 7: 13–31
14. Gowland C, Stratford P, Ward M, Moreland J, Torresin W, Van Hullenaar S, Sanford J, Barreca S, Vanspall B, Plews N (1993) Measuring physical impairment and disability with the Chedoke–McMaster stroke assessment. Stroke 24:58–63
15. Côté R, Battista RN, Wolfson C, Boucher J, Adam J, Hachinski V (1989) The Canadian neurological scale: validation and reliability assessment. Neurology 39:638–643
16. Brott T, Adams HP Jr, Olinger CP, Marler JR, Barsan WG, Biller J, Spilker J, Holleran R, Eberle R, Hertzberg V, Rorick M, Moomaw CJ, Walker M (1989) Measurements of acute cerebral infarction: a clinical examination scale. Stroke 20:864–870
17. Chino N, Sonoda S, Domen K, Saitoh E, Kimura A (1996) Stroke impairment assessment set (SIAS): In: Chino M, Melvin JL (eds) Functional evaluation of stroke patients. Springer, Tokyo, pp 19–31
18. Domen K (1995) Reliability and validity of stroke impairment assessment set (SIAS) (1) (in Japanese with English abstract). Jpn J Rehabil Med 32:113–122
19. Sonoda S (1995) Reliability and validity of stroke impairment assessment set (SIAS) (2): the items comprise the trunk, higher cortical function, and sensory function, and effectiveness as outcome predictor) (in Japanese with English abstract). Jpn J Rehabil Med 32:123–132

20. Gladman JRF, Harwood DMJ, Barer DH (1992) Predicting the outcome of acute stroke: prospective evaluation of five multivariate models and comparison with simple methods. J Neurol Neurosurg Psychiatry 55:347–351
21. Falconer JA, Naughton BJ, Dunlop DD, Roth EJ, Strasser DC, Sinacore JM (1994) Predicting stroke inpatient rehabilitation outcome using a classification tree approach. Arch Phys Med Rehabil 75:619–625
22. Granger CV, Hamilton BB, Linacre JM, Heinemann AW, Wright BD (1993) Performance profiles of the functional independence measure. Am J Phys Med Rehabil 72:84–89
23. Heinemann AW, Linacre JM, Wright BD, Hamilton BB, Granger CV (1993) Relationships between impairment and physical disability as measured by the Functional Independence Measure. Arch Phys Med Rehabil 74:566–573
24. Spitznagel EL, Helzer JE (1985) A proposed solution to the base rate problem in the kappa statistics. Arch Gen Psychiatry 42:725–728
25. Lincoln NB, Jackson JM, Edmans JA, Walker MF, Farrow VM, Latham A, Coombes K (1990) The accuracy of predictions about progress of patients on a stroke unit. J Neurol Neurosurg Psychiatry 53:972–975
26. Granger CV, Hamilton BB (1994) The uniform data system for medical rehabilitation report of first admissions for 1992. Am J Phys Med Rehabil 73:51–55

Advantages and Disadvantages of the Functional Independence Measure for Home Care

Tetsuya Adachi[1]

Summary. In Yokohama City, we have a visiting rehabilitation service system project for home patients. We have studied the validity of the Functional Independence Measure (FIM) data of 141 home patients. As the FIM raw score, an ordinal number, is difficult to quantify, efforts were made to convert the raw score to an interval measure. We attempted this conversion by using a quantification method of the third type. By this method we extracted factor 1, which indicates the independence ratings of the patients on the FIM items. We compared the results of the FIM data between inpatients and home patients. For home patients, the distribution pattern of the FIM items with respect to the independence ratings is easily affected by the environment around the patients. Thus, it is not easy to measure any quantitative change that is brought about by the changes of the environment of the patients. The FIM, by definition, contains two kinds of evaluation factors, one relating to the physical functions of the patients and the other to the environment surrounding the patients. Thus it is difficult to measure quantitative change of independence ratings of the FIM items for patients, especially for home patients who are sensitive to any changes in their surroundings.

Introduction

The functional independence measure (FIM) has been used in many countries since its establishment in 1983. We understand that tens of thousands of sample data have been stored in the Uniform Data Set (UDS). There have been many studies on the FIM using the UDS data in the United States, and several studies on the FIM have also been reported in Japan. We have used the FIM for inpatients and patients being cared for at home (hereafter referred to as "home patients") by referring to the UDS guidebook [1], videotape, and *UDS News*.

Many authors have reported on interrater and intrarater reliability and it appears that the reliability of the FIM is fairly well established. Granger and his colleagues have also reported on the validity of inpatient FIM data with many samples taken from the UDS and suggested that further studies are needed to solve problems concerning the FIM [2].

---

[1]Yokohama Municipal Citizens' Hospital, Okazawacho, Hodogayaku, Yokohama City 56, Japan

Although my experience with the validity of the FIM data of home patients is limited, I would like to discuss some of the problems associated with this subject.

Materials and Methods

Before discussing the validity of the FIM, I would like to mention the visiting rehabilitation service system for the home-bound physically disabled that was started in 1985 in Yokohama City, in which the subjects of this study were included.

In Yokohama City we have a visiting rehabilitation service system project for home patients to assist the patients and their families in maintaining the patients' capabilities, reducing the burden of care imposed on their families, and improving the quality of home life for these patients. In practice, a public health nurse refers a home patient who needs rehabilitative care to the rehabilitation center. Then, the rehabilitation team pays a first visit to the patient at home. This team consists of a physiatrist, a physical therapist or an occupational therapist, a public health nurse, and a social worker. From their joint analysis, we devise a program for improving or maintaining the patient's capability and improving or renovating the home environment. An appropriate team of staff visits the patient several times to implement the program and to determine whether the intended purpose has been achieved. The content of a typical rehabilitation program consists mainly of offering methods of performing the activities of daily living (ADL) by installing handrails, ensuring that floors are level, introducing some kind of assisting devices and tools, and providing house remodeling plans, and whatever else that may be necessary.

The study was carried out for 141 home patients who received visiting rehabilitation services, and the ADL was evaluated with the FIM between April 1991 and May 1992. The patients were those with brain dysfunction (61%), orthopedic impairment (12%), or neuromuscular diseases (11%).

We analyzed only 10 items related to motor functions of the FIM, excluding the following: bladder control, bowel control, stair climbing, and 5 items related to cognitive function (Table 1). We excluded the 5 items related to cognitive function and the 3 items related to motor function of the FIM because of information obtained from the report by Granger et al. [2]. They pointed out that the items related to motor and cognitive functions should be analyzed separately because they are of a different character. These researchers also noted that the items on bladder and bowel management provoke a statistical incompatability because they contain two different factors, continence and management. They also pointed out that the item of stair climbing shows statistical discrepancy: its score is affected by the fact that going up and down stairs is often not practiced for the sake of the patients' safety. The 10 items related to motor functions used for this study are shown on Table 1.

The FIM raw score, an ordinal number, is difficult to quantify, and thus some efforts were made to convert the raw score to an interval measure. In analyzing the results of rehabilitation by home visits, we attempted this conversion by using the quantification method of the third type. Each item of the FIM contains 7 categories; thus 10 items contain 70 categories. In our data conversion, we regarded each of these 70 categories as independent. We extracted factor 1, which had a high score of proper value of 0.73 (Table 2). The proper value is an index of accuracy about sample ordering on the dimensions of the extracted factor. The maximum proper value is 1.0.

Table 1. Ten motor items of the functional
independence measure (FIM).

1. Eating
2. Grooming
3. Bathing
4. Dressing upper body
5. Dressing lower body
6. Toileting
7. Toilet transfer
8. Tub transfer
9. Chair transfer
10. Walking
11. Bladder management
12. Bowel management
13. Stairs
14. Comprehension
15. Expression
16. Social interraction
17. Problem solving
18. Memory

Table 2. Proper value and category
scores of the FIM items calculated by the
quantification method of the third type
(70 categories).

Proper Value	Factor 1, 0.73	Factor 2, 0.51

Category scores

	Eating	Grooming	Bathing
1	0.039	0.032	0.018
2	0.039	0.033	−0.012
3	0.033	0.004	−0.021
4	0.026	0.009	−0.043
5	0.012	−0.000	−0.027
6	−0.007	−0.023	−0.043
7	−0.034	−0.044	−0.058

This high score of proper value of factor 1 suggests that the sample is well ordered on the dimensions of factor 1.

The distribution of the 70 categories is shown in Fig. 1. The figure indicates that factor 1 might be the one that shows the independence ratings of the patient in the 70 categories of the FIM.

Results

Figure 2 shows the category scores for each item of the FIM. I regarded factor 1 as the factor that indicates the independence ratings of the patient in the 70 categories. The

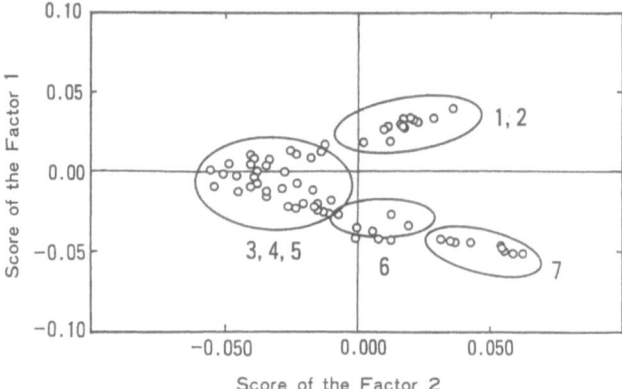

Fig. 1. Distribution of the 70 categories of the Functional Independence Measure (FIM). The *ordinate* represents the score of factor 1 and the *abscissa* the score of factor 2. Categories with higher levels of each of the FIM items are positioned in the lower portion on the ordinate, and categories with lower levels of each of the FIM items are positioned in the upper portion

scores of factor 1, which we call the converted FIM score, are regarded as the interval measure.

Figure 3 shows the calculations of the converted FIM score for each item of the home patients and of the inpatients. It can be seen that the home patient and inpatient calculations are almost linearly correlated. The six items lie along the identity line, while the other four items (bathing, dressing the upper body, chair transfer, and toilet transfer) are located a little farther from the line. AS to bathing and dressing the upper body, the home patients' independence ratings are lower than those of the inpatients.

Conversely, concerning chair and toilet transfers, the home patients' independence ratings are higher. It is believed that family members assist patients in bathing and dressing the upper body regardless of the patient's abilities; in other words, patients and their families do not feel strongly about independence when bathing and dressing the upper body are concerned. According to our experience, on the other hand, patients and their families both wish strongly for independence concerning chair and toilet transfers, so everyone makes an effort to be independent about such items. As a result, the independence ratings of the patient on these items increases, or, to put it another way, the degree by which the patient's need for independence with respect to the items will strongly affect the independence ratings on the FIM items.

Figure 4 shows the calculations of the converted FIM scores on each item of home patients before and after rehabilitation services. Note that the home patients' calculations before and after rehabilitation services are almost linearly correlated. The seven items lie along the identity line, while the other three items, chair, toilet, and tub transfers, are located slightly away from these seven items. For these three items, the calculations that show independence ratings improved after rehabilitation services more than those for the other seven items. This occurred because our home visit rehabilitation services have been designed mainly for improving the transfer capability, and resulted in changing the distribution pattern of the FIM items with respect to the independence ratings after the rehabilitation intervention. Figure 5, from Granger et al. [2], shows the calculations of the FIM items at admission and discharge. Note that admission and discharge calculations are similar.

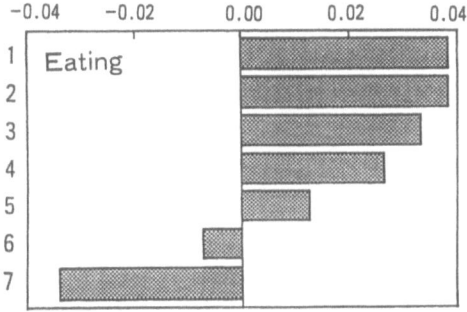

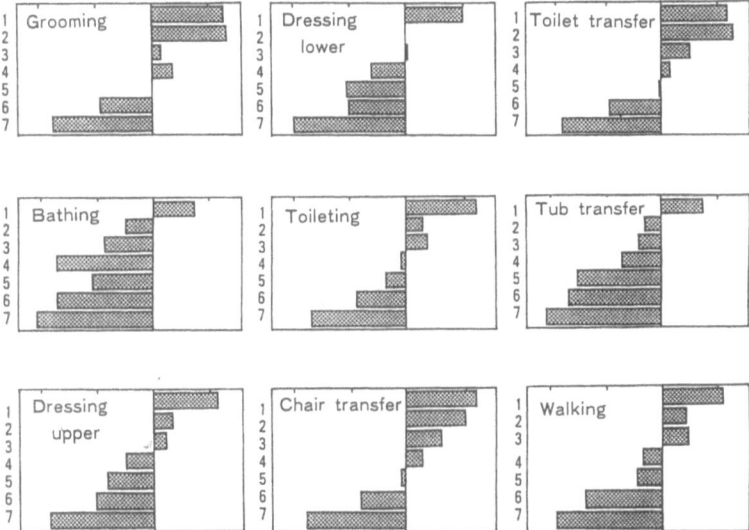

Fig. 2. Category scores of FIM items. Scores shown for "eating" are ordered according to the seven-level classification of the FIM. Scores for the other nine items are ordered in the same way

By means of the rehabilitation programs in the medical facilities, recovery of the physical functions of the inpatients directly resulted in an improvement in the independence ratings for all the FIM items. Thus, the distribution pattern of the FIM items with respect to the independence ratings of the inpatients has not changed by the rehabilitation program. For home patients, however, a change of the environment around the patient has a strong effect on the independence ratings of the FIM items, and this effect has been reflected only in the specific FIM items such as bathing and chair and toilet transfers. Thus, a change of the environment around the patient may have a considerable effect on the distribution pattern of the FIM items with respect to the independence ratings.

Figure 6 shows the number of patients whose independence rating has improved after home visit rehabilitation as ascertained by the FIM raw score and the Barthel index. Based on the FIM raw scores, improvements were found in 108 of 141 patients (76.6%), and based on the Barthel index, in 28 of 141 patients (19.9%). It seems that

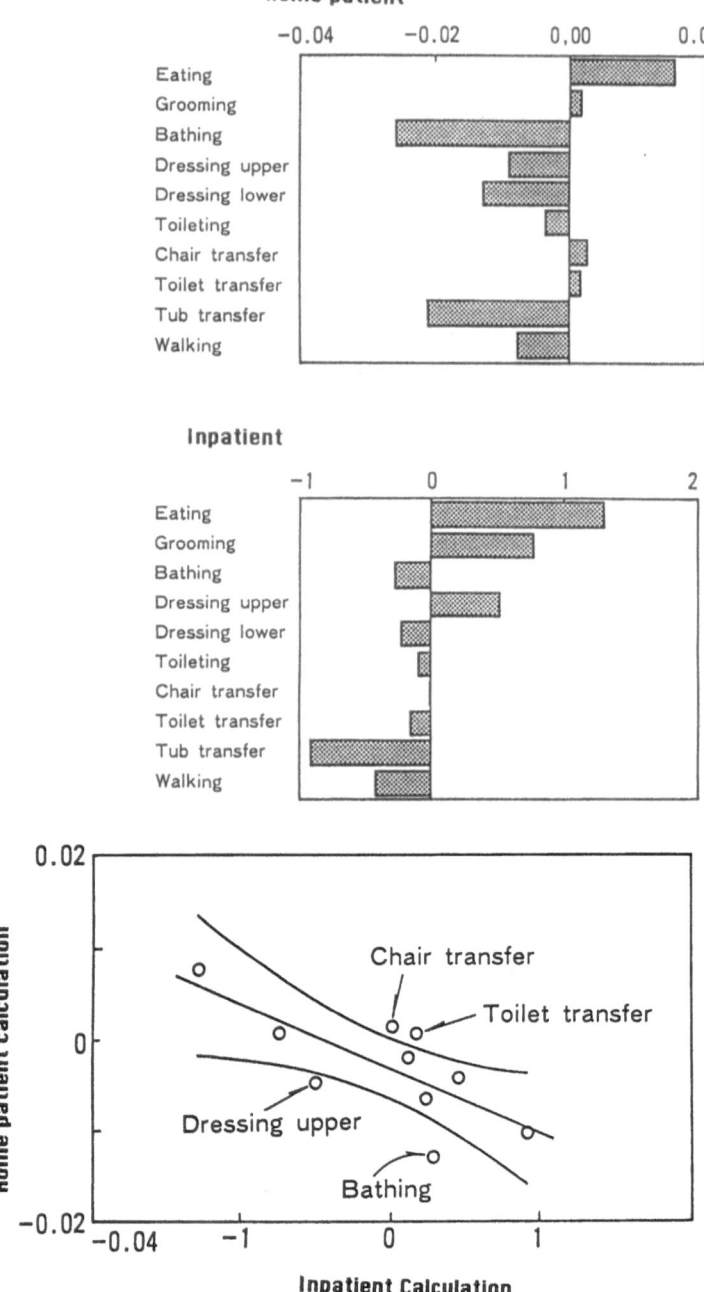

Fig. 3. Calculations of converted FIM score items for home patients and inpatients. Calculations for home patients (*top panel*) have been converted by the quantification method of the third type; calculations for inpatients (*middle panel*) have been converted by Rasch analysis. The *bottom panel* shows the relationship between the calculations for home patients (*ordinate*) and inpatients (*abscissa*)

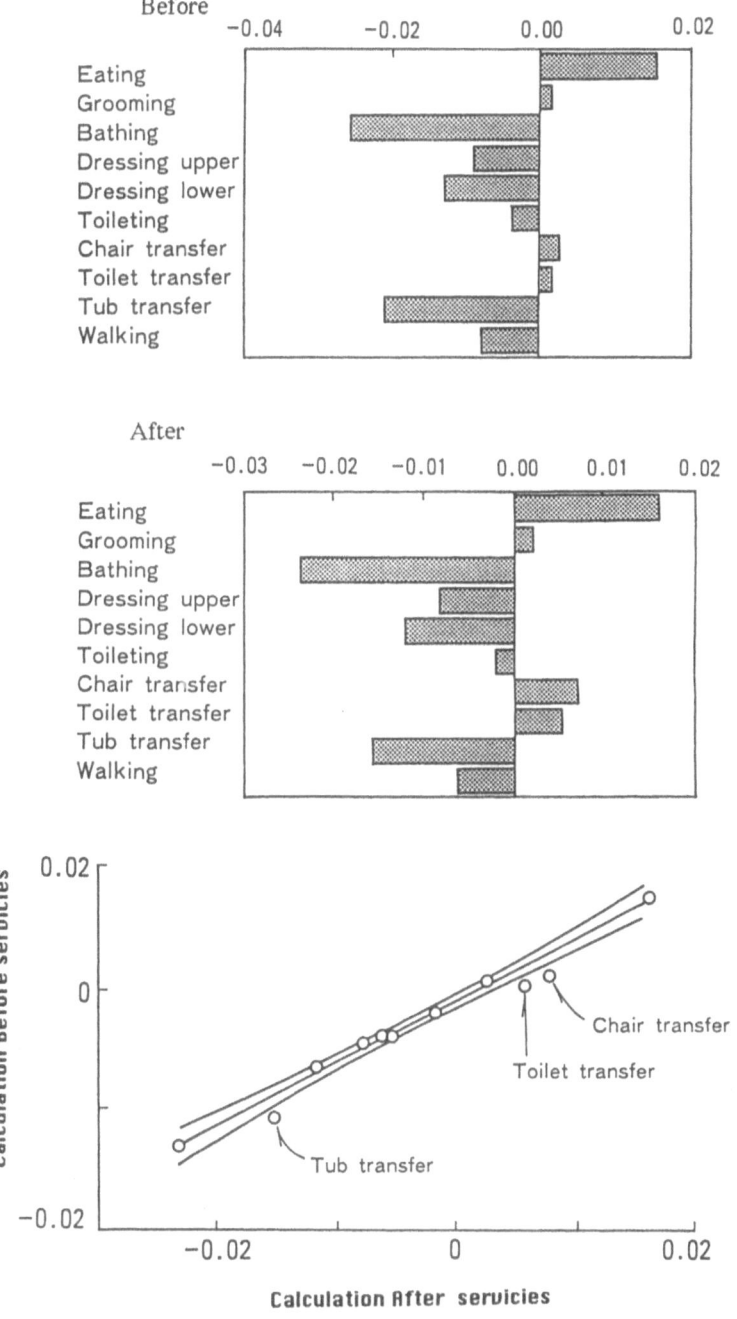

Fig. 4. Calculations of converted FIM score items for home patients and inpatients before (*top*) and after (*middle*) rehabilitation services. The bottom panel shows the relationship between calculations for home patients before and after rehabilitation services

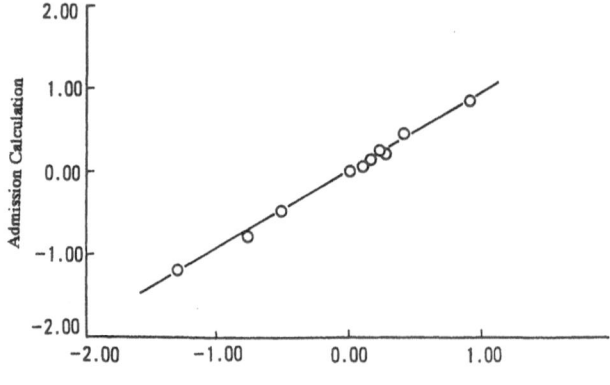

Fig. 5. Calculations of FIM items at admission and discharge. (From [2], with permission)

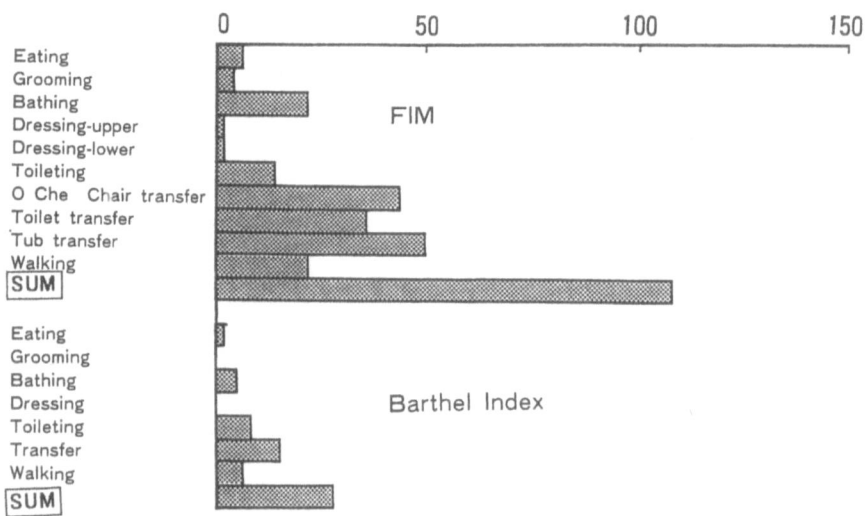

Fig. 6. Number of patients whose independence ratings has improved after home visit rehabilitation

the FIM is more sensitive and useful than the Barthel index for the assessment of the ADL independence in the home visit rehabilitation of severely handicapped patients.

Conclusion

1. The distribution patterns of the FIM items with respect to the independence ratings by the interval measure are slightly different when comparing home patients and inpatients. This may be because the need of the patient and his family for independence as related to these items markedly affects the independence ratings of the FIM items at home. It seems that in dressing and bathing, Japanese families customarily assist patients. On the other hand, transfer activities require considerable physical assistance and it is desired that patients regain independence.

2. On the home visit rehabilitation program, we not only offer instructions for gaining better functional activity but also recommend and assist in modifying the environment around the patients, such as employing transfer devices and remodeling the house. This makes a difference in the distribution patterns of the FIM items with respect to the independence ratings of the home patients before and after rehabilitation services.

3. To measure the quantitative change of each FIM item, the distribution pattern of the FIM items with respect to the independence ratings of the patients must be constant. For inpatients, the distribution pattern is constant at admission and discharge; for home patients, the distribution pattern is easily affected by the change of the environment surrounding the patients. Thus it is not easy to measure any quantitative change that is brought about by changes of the environment.

4. A change of the physical functions of the patients affects all the FIM items in a relatively similar manner. On the other hand, a change of the environment affects only specific items. Thus, a change of the physical function does not affect the distribution pattern of the FIM items but a change of the environment does affect the distribution pattern.

The FIM, by definition, contains two kinds of evaluation factors: one relating to the physical functions and the other to the environment around the patients. Thus it is difficult to measure the quantitative change of the independence ratings of the FIM items, especially of home patients, who are sensitive to any changes of the environment around themselves.

References

1. Granger CV, Hamilton BB, Shelwin FS (1986) Guide for use of the uniform data set for medical rehabilitation. Buffalo General Hospital, Buffalo
2. Linacare JM, Heinemann AW, Wright BB, Granger CV, Hamilton BB (1994) The structure and stability of the functional independence measure. Arch Phys Med Rehabil 75:127–132

Toward Future Research

Meigen Liu[1] and Shigenobu Ishigami[2]

Summary. Stroke is the number-one disability group with regard to patient numbers and the impact upon health care systems. To improve our management skills and the quality of rehabilitation programs, we need to evaluate our patients objectively and predict their functional outcomes as early and as accurately as possible. In this chapter, the methodological problems related to stroke outcome research and directions for the future are discussed. We need to develop a valid and reliable set of standardized measures of stroke pathology, comorbidity, impairment, disability, handicap, and life satisfaction that could be uniformly and internationally used. Future studies should follow well-designed and standardized protocols including patient selection, measures used, acquisition, management, and analysis of data so that different studies could be compared and conclusions generalized. In addition, international cooperative research would provide us with an unique opportunity to acquire further insight into the problems related to stroke rehabilitation, and refinement of the methodology in this area is needed.

Introduction

With increasing populations of elderly persons in Japan, the United States, and European countries, we are faced with enormous medical and welfare problems that demand urgent solutions. Under stringent economic conditions, we must formulate strategies to efficiently allocate the limited medical and welfare resources so that we can enhance the quality of life of the disabled and at the same time minimize the burden of care to society. To achieve these goals, we need to objectively measure the impact of disabling illness on our society.

It is also important for rehabilitation professionals in various countries to exchange information, share experiences, cooperatively analyze problems, and work together for policy making concerning medical care and welfare systems for the disabled. To

[1] Department of Rehabilitation Medicine, Saitama Prefecture General Rehabilitation Center, 148-1 Nishikaizuka, Ageo City, Saitama 361, Japan, and Department of Rehabilitation Medicine, Keio University School of Medicine, 35-Shinanomachi, Shinjyuku-ku, Tokyo 160, Japan
[2] Department of Rehabilitation Medicine, National Defense Medical College, 3-2 Namiki, Tokorozawa City, Saitama 359, Japan

facilitate this type of international cooperation, it is indispensable for us to have a common language or measures of the three aspects of disablement (impairment, disability, and handicap), as defined by the World Health Organization [1], and to formulate a common framework for outcome studies of disabling illness. In this respect, the Uniform Data System (UDS) is the first and the largest rehabilitation database to cover the United States as well as several other countries in the world [2]. It allows us, for the first time, to compare outcome data internationally using a uniform measure of disability, the Functional Independence Measure (FIM), and a standardized format of data collection.

Based on UDS data, important outcome studies concerning medical rehabilitation are emerging [3,4]. The UDS, however, has the limitations in that data collected are confined to demographic data, disability as measured with FIM, placement, and insurance. So far not much attention has been paid to the aspects of pathology, comorbidity, and impairment, with the exception of spinal cord injury in which the American Spinal Injury Association's Standards of Neurological Classification (ASIA) [5] are utilized as a part of the UDS to describe impairment.

Among the disabling conditions, stroke is the number-one disability group with regard to patient number and the impact upon health care and welfare systems with which we as rehabilitation professionals must contend in our daily practice [6]. In Japan, for example, stroke was the most frequent cause of death until 1981 [7]. Currently it is the third most frequent cause of death, following cancer and cardiac diseases. The mortality rate was 96.2 per 100 000 in 1991. In contrast, the rate of stroke patients receiving medical care has increased from 118 per 100 000 in 1970 to 305 per 100 000 in 1991. This increase can mostly be explained by an increase in the number of inpatient stroke patients. In 1991, the number of disabled persons was estimated as 2 722 000, and among them, 325 000 (11.9%) were stroke patients [7].

To improve our clinical management skills and the quality of our rehabilitation programs while making the best use of limited resources, we must be able to evaluate our patients objectively and predict their functional outcomes as early and as accurately as possible. Detailed review and updating of functional evaluation and prognostication, as well as presentations of newer ideas and ongoing research, are given in other chapters of this monograph. The purposes of this final chapter are to review the methodological problems related to outcome studies and to point out directions for future research.

Methodological Problems Related to Outcome Studies

The objectives of stroke outcome research are prognostication, evaluation of therapeutic efficacy, program evaluation, and health care planning. Although there have been many outcome studies of stroke patients, most of them are fraught with at least one of the following shortcomings [8,9]: (1) lack of specification of selection criteria and characteristics of the patient population studied; (2) lack of use of standardized assessment and outcome measures that have proven validity and reliability; (3) lack of specification of the study design, including timing and method of data collection; (4) lack of information concerning the therapeutic interventions provided; (5) lack of proper use of statistical methods for data analysis; and (6) lack of cross-validation and multicenter trials. These problems make it difficult to compare various outcome studies or apply the prediction rules developed in one study to other population samples. It is therefore essential to formulate a valid working model for future outcome studies.

In this connection, the recommendations released at the Symposium on Methodological Issues in Stroke Outcome Research [10] should be the basis for future research designing. In essence, the Task Forces on Impairment, Disability and Handicap made the following 14 recommendations.

1. Time points from onset of stroke should be used.
2. Laterality should refer to the side of the brain lesion.
3. The entire study population should be classified by a single imaging technique.
4. Study population should be limited to patients with initial stroke.
5. Strokes should be classified by type and location.
6. The recommended time intervals for sequential observations are onset, 3, 6, and 12 months.
7. Disability scales should include the domains of self-care activities, locomotion, sphincter control, communications, cognition, and behavior.
8. Disability assessment should be based on performance, not on capacity.
9. Disability should be related to specific impairments.
10. Outcome variables should include survival, place of residence, living arrangements, change in activities of daily living (ADL), change in complex instrumental ADL (IADL), change in social function, utilization of health care resources, satisfaction with life, and ability to work.
11. Research literature on stroke handicap needs to be synthesized.
12. New research instruments for the study of stroke handicap need to be developed.
13. Context of stroke handicap should be included.
14. Handicap before and after stroke should be detailed.

Similarly, the recent accomplishments of Patient Outcomes Research Teams (PORTs) are also suggestive for future research [11]. PORTs are groups of investigators involved in 14 special outcome studies including ischemic heart disease, childbirth, low birthweight, pneumonia, biliary tract disease, cataract management, and so on. Each of the PORTs has followed a standard research model involving the application of systematic literature review, measurement of outcomes, analysis of cost and claims data, decision analysis, and strategies for disseminating findings. Through collaborative work of inter-PORT work groups, PORTs have contributed significantly to methodological advances in outcome research. They are providing a previously unavailable opportunity to assess different outcomes research projects through meetings, conferences and publications.

The issues that have been studied by PORT work groups are (1) question selection and design, (2) research design, (3) data collection, and (4) data interpretation [12]. The outcome measures include survival, morbidity, complications, physical functioning, and resource use (cost, readmissions), as well as "softer" outcomes such as overall health status, symptom relief, role functioning, and satisfaction with care [11]. Because well-designed outcome studies demand concerted efforts of experts from multiple disciplines, such as physicians, rehabilitation professionals, statisticians, and administrators, and efforts that are often beyond the capability of one individual, systematic peer review processes as practiced by PORT work groups will significantly contribute to the refinement of research design.

In this section, some of the problems that we encounter in designing outcome studies are discussed.

Measures

For measures to become clinically and scientifically meaningful, they must posses the following properties: validity, reliability, scalability, sensitivity, specificity, sensibility, and practicality [13–16]. In addition, a measure must be equipped with an adequate manual to ensure proper administration [14]. These requirements for measures are summarized in Table 1. Construction of a scale should follow established psychometric principles and statistical concepts regarding the types of scales (ratio, interval, ordinal, and nominal) [13]. For ordinal scales that are frequently used in rehabilitation medicine, sophisticated statistical methods such as Rasch analysis have been explored in recent years [17,18]. Rasch analysis allows one to position items according

Table 1. Requirements for the measures.

Items	Description	Methods of analysis
Validity	(1) The extent to which a test procedure measures what it purports to measure; (2) refers to the appropriateness, meaningfulness, and usefulness of a measure and of the inferences made from it	
Content validity	The degree to which a scale contains the items that represent the domain of interest	Face validity (expert opinion), factor analysis, Rasch analysis, cluster analysis
Criterion validity (predictive validity)	The extent to which a measure is related to a logically important outcome criterion	Regression analysis, discriminant analysis
Concurrent validity	The degree to which a measure is related to other events occurring at the same time	Correlation with other established measures; sensitivity and specificity
Construct validity	Tested by seeing whether a measure displays a pattern of converging relationship (convergent validity) and an absence of confounding relationship (divergent validity)	Multitrait–multimethod matrix, confirmatory factor analysis
Reliability	Defined as the degree to which a measure is free from random error	
Interrater reliability	The degree to which a measure, in the hands of one trained individual, gives the same result when used by other individuals	Kappa statistics, intraclass correlation coefficient
Test–retest reliability	The degree to which a measure is consistent or reproducible when readministered by trained staff in maximally similar circumstances	Kappa statistics, intraclass correlation coefficient

Table 1. *Contuined.*

Items	Description	Methods of analysis
Internal consistency, unidimensionality	The items must (1) progress hierarchically from easy to difficult across the range of patient performance; (2) clearly define a common underlying trait or ability; (3) maintain a constant difficulty order for all patients	Split-half correlations, Cronbach alpha, factor analysis, Rasch analysis
Responsiveness	The ability to reflect important changes	
Sensitivity	The ability to detect the problem correctly	True-positive rate, false-negative rate
Specificity	The ability to avoid falsely labeling individuals who do not have the problem as having it	True-negative rate, false-positive rate
Sensibility, practicality	The reasonableness of using a measure	Determined by an important purpose for its inclusion and relative ease of its use

This table is based on studies by Nunnally and Bernstein [13], Johnston and Keith [14], and Silverstein et al. [15].

to difficulty and persons according to ability with regard to the items on a common unidimensional and additive scale, thus enabling one to handle ordinal scales just like interval scales and analyze the structure of the scales [18].

Care must be taken that measures whose validity and reliability are claimed on the basis of studies performed in certain population samples and under certain circumstances do not necessarily prove valid and reliable in different samples or settings [16]. This holds particularly true when a measure is used in international studies in which racial and sociocultural differences could be great.

Quite a large number of measures have been proposed so far for stroke evaluation; for a detailed review of this topic, the readers are referred to other chapters of this monograph or recently published books on measures [16,19]. Surprisingly, Jongbloed [8] noted, in his review of 33 studies, that 63% of these used scales whose reliability and validity are unknown. To make the outcome studies valid and comparable, it is advisable to use standardized measures as much as possible. To review and analyze various measures so far published, the standard format of the reviewing process proposed by Wilkin et al. [16] is helpful. This format consists of the purpose, background, description, administration, acceptability, reliability, validity, populations, and/or service settings in which a measure was developed plus general comments. There is currently an urgent need to develop a set of standardized measures for stroke outcome studies that could be used uniformly throughout the country as well as internationally. A brief review of measures for each category follows.

Pathology

Instead of lumping stroke patients together into the general term "stroke," it is important to classify them on the basis of information about the etiology, location, nature, and severity of stroke. Standard physical and neurological examinations coupled with neuroimaging techniques and other laboratory studies are necessary. As Kinkel [20] has recommended, the neuroimaging study for stroke outcome research should be done in the more chronic stage, preferably 1 month after onset when the findings are usually stabilized. It is also necessary to use a single method of neuroimaging, either computed tomography (CT) or magnetic resonance imaging (MRI), for a particular series of studies. A system for interpreting neuroimages by identifying the specific patterns of regional arterial ischemic infarction is proposed for CT and MRI [21,22], but no uniform method of reporting and coding the findings is available yet. It is necessary to develop a standard format of describing neuroimage findings.

Comorbidity

There are two types of comorbidity [10]. The first type includes those conditions that could compromise an individual's ability to function optimally, such as arthritis and other orthopedic problems, cardiopulmonary problems (ischemic heart disease, valvular heart disease, respiratory insufficiency, etc.), hearing and visual problems, metabolic and endocrine problems (obesity, diabetes mellitus, hepatic disorders, renal disorders, and so on), and psychiatric and neurological problems (depression, coexisting neurological disorders, etc.). The second type includes those conditions that have prognostic significance as risk factors of stroke, such as heart disease, diabetes mellitus, hypertension, and hyperlipidemia. These comorbid conditions could significantly influence the outcomes, but standardized measures of comorbidity are lacking. The Charlson Comorbidity Index [23] is one of the few validated indices available at this moment. This index is based upon actual mortality rates, assigning weighted values to comorbid conditions. The scale was validated in acute hospital settings, not in rehabilitation settings; it focuses on mortality, not on functional impairment, and the number of comorbid conditions is limited. There is an urgent need to develop a standardized comorbidity index applicable to rehabilitation patients so that we can stratify them according to comorbid conditions in outcome analysis.

Impairment

There are a host of measures of stroke impairment, either comprehensive [the Stroke Impairment Assessment Set (SIAS) [24], for example] or for specific impairment (Motricity index [25] for motor impairment, Ashworth Scale [26] for spasticity, and so on). The authors have been using the SIAS as developed by Chino and his group [24]. It is based on the recommendations of the Symposium on Methodological Issues in Stroke Outcome Research [10] and is a simple, comprehensive, reliable, sensitive, and valid assessment set of stroke impairment measures. The details of SIAS and how it can contribute to stroke outcome studies are covered in other chapters of this monograph. Thus far, not much attention has been paid to impairment as compared to disability in stroke outcome studies, and this is partly because of the lack of standardized measures of impairment. In this sense, SIAS would potentially be an useful instrument of stroke impairment for future studies.

Disability

Among the many measures of ADL available, the FIM is currently the most sophisticated. It fulfills most of the requirements for measures depicted in Table 1, and, particularly noteworthy, is the only measure so far developed that has a system to assure uniformity through a guidebook, videos, FIM letters, seminars, workshops, and a credentialing process. Another important advantage is that it provides a feedback system between the developers and users (FIM fax, teleconference, etc.) so that necessary improvements and refinement can continuously be made. In addition, through the recent studies of our group, its transcultural validity has been confirmed.

Using Rasch analysis, Tsuji et al. [27] analyzed the structure of FIM in Japanese stroke patients and compared it to that reported in U.S. patients. It was found that FIM could be separated into two subgroups of 13 motor FIM items and 5 cognitive FIM items as in the U.S. patients, and the mean square fit statistics (MNSQ), which indicates each item's adherence to the Rasch model restrictions concerning scale unidimensionality, was below 1.2 except for stair climbing, with a standard error of the measure of the order of 0.01 logits. The pattern of item difficulties was almost identical between the two countries, except for bowel and bladder management, which was easier for patients in Japan, and bathing and tub transfer, which were more difficult for Japanese patients. These differences could reasonably be explained by cultural differences. For example, Japanese are not satisfied only with taking a shower and would want to soak neck-deep in a unique, deep bathtub, making tub transfer and bathing more difficult as compared to Westerners.

In addition to basic ADL, measures for instrumental ADL (IADL) that include meal preparation, use of telephone, home maintenance, money management, ability to use transportation, ability to self-administer medication, shopping, and the like also need to be developed [10].

Handicap and Quality of Life

The dimensions of handicap include occupation, social integration, economic self-sufficiency, and family functioning. The Craig Handicap Assessment and Reporting Technique (CHART) [28], Life Satisfaction Index [LSI] [29], and Measure of Satisfaction (MOS) 36-Item Short-Form Health Survey (SF-36) [30] are some of the measures of handicap or quality of life [QOL] with evidence to support their reliability and validity. It is conceivable that sociocultural differences would play a very important role in the areas of handicap and QOL, and whether these standardized measures used in Western cultures could be used in other countries with different sociocultural backgrounds remains to be proved by future research.

Outcome Measures

In health science, outcome is usually defined in terms of the achievement of or failure to achieve desired goals [16]. Sometimes a change in functional status (gain) over a specified time period is used to measure outcome. As pointed out by Cronbach et al. [31], however, raw gain scores obtained by subtracting pretest scores from posttest scores could lead to fallacious conclusions because such scores are systematically related to any random error of measurement. To measure outcome, the following indices are used either singularly or in combination: survival, reattack of stroke, functional gain (motor recovery, functional improvement etc., over the study period), functional outcome (state of disability at a specified time), discharge disposition, length of hospital stay, resource utilization, cost, life satisfaction, and social functioning [10,11,16]. It would be desirable to develop a set of standard outcome measures for each category of pathology, impairment, disability, handicap, and QOL, and synthesize them to form a composite scale that could represent total rehabilitation outcome. In this respect the study by Falconer et al. [32] is suggestive. They defined favorable outcome as meeting the three criteria of discharge to community (handicap), survival greater than 3 months post discharge (pathology), and no more than minimal physical assistance in functional activities (disability).

Research Design and Data Analysis

Selection of Patient Population

To make a study comparable to others and the conclusions general in application, the criteria for patient selection should be clearly stated. Demographic data including gender, age, race, socioeconomic status (social class, marital status, educational level, employment, etc.) are necessary. Information concerning the etiology, type and severity of stroke as well as comorbidity is also important [8]. The sample size preferably should be large, and the characteristics of the sample as compared to the general population should be stated. To minimize the effect of confounding factors and to facilitate analysis of the causal relationship between variables and outcomes, the study population should be stratified by stroke mechanism, severity of stroke, comorbidity, demographic data, facility, and treatment as much as possible [12]. Multicenter trials are preferred to avoid selection bias.

Specification of the Study Design

Information as to the timing and methods of measurement is essential. As pointed out by Jongbloed [8], there are hazards in using events such as discharge rather than time post stroke as markers in measuring stroke recovery. In future studies, it is important to measure patient function at set times post stroke. In addition, previous studies have usually failed to specify the kind of therapy the patients are receiving during the study period. Information is necessary regarding the acute phase therapy for stroke, both medical and surgical, the time interval from onset to admission to rehabilitation services, criteria for entry into the program, and timing, duration, frequency, quantity, and type of exercise [8].

Database

Because data collected in rehabilitation medicine are multifaceted and numerous, it is indispensable to develop a systematic, well-organized database to facilitate clinical management and research. With ever-improving computer technology and software, it is recently far easier to develop a database. There are many isolated databases effective only for a particular individual, department, facility, or study group, but there was none that was universally applicable until the development of UDS [2].

The UDS was started in 1987 and is the world's first comprehensive and large-scale national registry of standardized information on medical rehabilitation, covering almost half the U.S. rehabilitation facilities and several facilities in other countries. It collects data on each patient's age, gender, living situation before hospitalization, diagnosis leading to disability, time since onset of disability, and functional status at admission and discharge. The mission of the UDS is establishment and maintenance of disability and outcome measures, collection, management, and analysis of data, feedback to the subscribers, and research [2]. It is growing year by year and is continuously refined by incorporating newer developments in functional assessment, such as ASIA for spinal cord injury [5] and Function-Related Groups (FRGs) for length of stay estimation [33], and by developing sophisticated software called FIMware [34].

Although this kind of systematized and uniform database is no doubt indispensable for improving medical rehabilitation, it does not necessarily suit the individual needs of each facility or a particular study group and thus there is also a need for a customized database. Many researchers are developing their own databases. For example, the Keio Rehabilitation Data System (KRDS) has been used since 1991 for everyday clinical management and research at the Department of Rehabilitation Medicine, Keio University School of Medicine, and its affiliated facilities. It is a personal computer-based, clinically and research-oriented, user-friendly, easily customizable database that incorporates standardized measures (SIAS, FIM, Mini-Mental State Test, etc.), and is capable of graphically displaying patient impairment, disability profile, and progress.

The system was originally developed by Domen and Liu, and went through several modifications and refinements through clinical use. It consists of several files (Fig. 1); all the information, once input, can be used to produce a conference sheet, a patient progress summary, administrative files, patient and family education materials, and a discharge summary. Equations to predict the probability of FIM level 6 and 7 of ambulation and total discharge FIM scores from variables measured on admission have been incorporated into the system, facilitating patient management significantly. There are or will be many of these kinds of stand-alone databases throughout the world, and there will surely be a need to link these individualized, customized

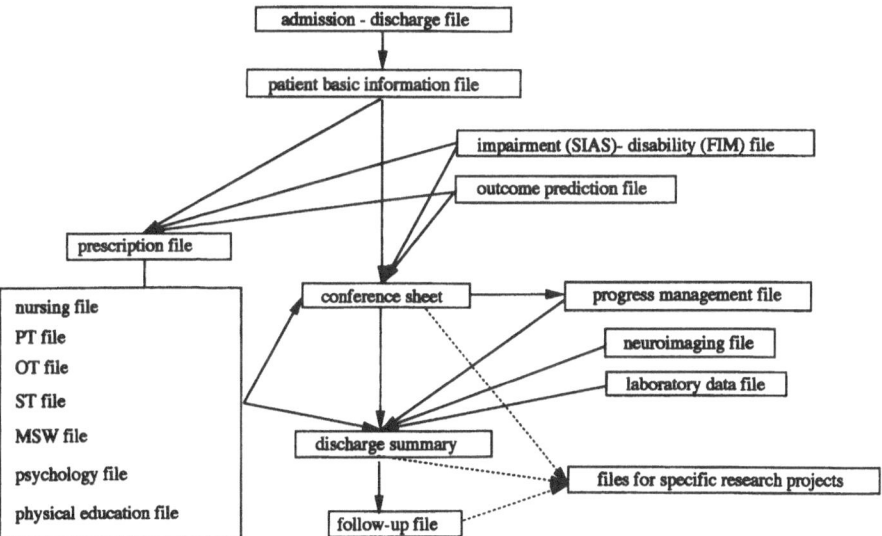

Fig. 1. The Keio Rehabilitation Data System (KRDS) is a personal computer (Macintosh, Apple Computer Inc.) based database that consists of the files depicted in the figure. It is oriented toward daily clinical management and research, especially outcome research. SIAS, stroke impairment assessment set; FIM, functional independence measure; PT, physical therapy; OT, occupational therapy; ST, speech therapy; MSW, medical social worker

databases to a large scale, uniform database like UDS in the future. To promote international research, some guidelines will be necessary with regard to database development to assure compatibility and to maintain uniformity. In the process, problems concerning intellectual properties of the measures, software, or databases developed may also need to be resolved.

Data Analysis

Various statistical methods, from the simplest to the most sophisticated and sometimes complicated, have been used in outcome studies. Statistical methods when used properly can help to design trials, clarify the causal relationship between various clinical factors and outcomes, and enable us to predict what can be achieved through rehabilitation programs. Unfortunately, because of the complexity of statistical methods and unfamiliarity with them on the part of most clinicians, usually not enough consideration has been given when designing a study and selecting methods of data analysis.

Because these are very important aspects of determining the quality of research, it is desirable to consult medical statisticians or experts in clinical trials when formulating a protocol of an outcome study. The authors sincerely wish that this issue would be formally addressed by experts involved in outcomes research as a task force to make recommendations and general guidelines for research design and data analysis. In addition to written guidelines, an interactive software program that a clinician attempting an outcome study can use to check the protocol, something similar to the system described by Wyatt et al. [35], would be helpful. It is beyond the capability of the authors to discuss the full scope of research design and data analysis, but we would like to review methods commonly used in outcomes research and point out several problems encountered in outcomes studies from the clinicians' point of view.

Stratification

As stated earlier, stratification of the study population by stroke mechanism, severity of stroke, comorbidity, demographic data, facility, treatment options, and so on is necessary to minimize the effect of confounding factors. After stratification, simpler statistics such as the repeated chi-square method or the Mantel–Haenszel method can be used. Usually, however, a large sample is needed to adjust for all the confounding factors. When the number of cases is limited and confounding factors are multiple, differences between groups are not easily detected because the sample size for each subgroup becomes too small. In this situation, multivariate analysis is more appropriate [36].

Multivariate Analysis

Multivariate analysis is useful when the sample size is relatively small and still the variables that could influence prognosis are multiple. With this method, it is possible to weigh the contribution of each variable to outcome measures considering multiple variables together. There are several methods of multivariate analysis, and appropriate methods should be chosen based on the purpose of the analysis and characteristics of the variables (Table 2). In Western literature, there has been a tendency to use multiple regression analysis or discriminant analysis even when the variables are ordinal, but theoretically this could be misleading. For ordinal variables, quantification theory type 1 or type 2 developed by Hayashi [37] is more appropriate. A newer

Table 2. Methods of multivariate analysis.

Method	Criterion variable	Explanatory variable	Objectives
Multiple regression analysis	Single interval scale	Multiple interval scales	Predict a criterion variable from multiple interval scales
Multiple logistic model	Single interval scale (0–1)	Multiple interval scales	Predict a criterion variable (0–1) from multiple interval scales
Discriminant analysis	Two or more groups	Multiple interval scales	Discriminate groups from multiple interval scales
Quantification method 1	Single interval scale	Multiple ordinal scales	Predict a criterion variable from multiple ordinal scales
Quantification method 2	Two or more groups	Multiple ordinal scales	Discriminate groups from multiple ordinal scales
Piecewise regression	Single interval scale	Multiple interval scales	Divide the regression equation into two parts
Conversational data analysis	Single interval or ordinal scale	Multiple interval and/or ordinal scales	Analyze interactively data set that includes both interval and ordinal data
Principal component analysis	None	Multiple interval or ordinal scales	Represent multiple variables by a single or a few variable(s) without losing information, and summarize multiple variables
Canonical correlation analysis	Multiple interval or ordinal scales	Multiple interval scales	Correlate groups of criteria and explanatory variables
Factor analysis	None	Multiple interval scales	Explain the information of various variables by a few common factors
Cluster analysis	None	Multiple interval scales	Classify into clusters by compiling factors according to similarity

method called Conversational Data Analysis (CSA), developed by Haga [38] enables a researcher to analyze interactively a data set that includes both interval and categorical data, so that he or she can handle both types of data collectively and integrate multiple regression analysis, discriminant analysis, and quantification theories. The selection of explanatory variables is achieved interactively with the computer program. This method was successfully used by Domen et al. [39] to predict motor FIM scores from impairment variables measured with SIAS.

Another method of multivariate analysis often used in prognostication studies is logistic regression. It is a mathematical modeling approach that can be used to describe the relationship of several independent variables to a dichotomous dependent variable [40]. The logistic function on which the model is based provides estimates that must lie in the range between zero and one and an S-shaped description of the combined effect of several risk factors on the risk for a disease. The probability that an individual would develop the disease or certain consequences (becoming ambulatory, etc.) over some defined follow-up time interval can be obtained.

Classification Tree Analysis

Multivariate analysis has been extensively used in recent outcome studies, but according to Falconer et al. [32], prediction models commonly used in outcome studies have the following problems: (1) they generally characterize one outcome (i.e., functional status, discharge disposition, costs) whereas the clinician must consider all outcomes; (2) they identify the predictor variables and may include interaction terms but do not delineate the interactions among predictor variables; (3) the results are usually expressed as regression coefficients, explained variance, and P values, which have no intuitive correlate to the clinical decision; and (4) traditional regression methods are undesirable to use with functional status variables because of the ordinal nature of the data and the difficulty in interpreting traditional regression coefficients when applied to variables with unequal intervals.

Considering these limitations of traditional multivariate analysis, Falconer et al. proposed using a classification tree approach (CART), a nonparametric analysis that can handle variables with unequal intervals, to develop a set of decision rules for the prediction of global outcome. To predict favorable rehabilitation outcome, which they defined as meeting the three criteria of discharge to community, survival for more than 3 months post discharge, and no more than minimal physical assistance in functional activities, they first developed a large classification tree through a series of binary splits. The procedures consisted of (1) systematic evaluation of all potential divisions of a predictor variable to find the best division that separates the favorable from the unfavorable outcomes; (2) repetition of this process for all the remaining predictor variables; (3) selection of the predictor variables that best separate the outcomes; and (4) pruning of the large tree to a smaller, more efficient tree by striking a balance between the tree size and the overall classification error that is assessed by a cross-validation technique [32,41]. All these procedures are performed fully automatically with the aid of sophisticated software [42]. Using this method, they identified four predictor variables of toilet management, bladder management, toilet transfer, and adequacy of financial resources with a prediction accuracy of 88% and a cross-validation error rate of 18%.

Another successful application of CART is a study reported by Stineman et al. [33]. In their study of 39 680 patients enrolled in UDS, they developed the Function Related

Groups (FRGs) to predict length of stay (LOS) using only four predictor variables: impairment category, motor and cognitive FIM scores at time of admission, and age. The classification method was based on recursive-partitioning classification and regression trees. The LOS variance explained by linear regression was 32.9% in the analysis and 31.3% in the validation data sample [33].

The CART is a different way to expand the scope of linear regression, and it differs from classical predecessors in that it substitutes computer algorithms for the traditional mathematical ways of getting numerical answers, and requires fewer distributional assumptions [43]. It can handle ordinal data and readily identifies the interactions among predictor variables; also, the results are easily communicated [32]. Improved algorithms for CART have been reported [44,45]. It is a promising data analysis tool for future outcome research.

Life-Table Analysis

Reding [46] used life-table analysis to predict the probability of ambulation. The Barthel index was measured prospectively at 2-week intervals, and the probability of walking more than 150 ft without assistance was plotted for each subgroup of patients (motor deficit only; motor and sensory deficit; and motor, sensory, and visual deficit) and compared using the Mantel–Haenszel log-rank method. With life-table analysis, it is possible to use observation periods of all cases even if they are different for each individual [47]. The observational periods are divided into certain lengths, and probability of a certain endpoint (in the example just cited, the probability of walking) is plotted for each study group and compared. The method has the advantages that it can provide data for setting patient rehabilitation goals, indicate otherwise unrecognized comorbid medical-behavioral problems, and allow comparing the effect of rehabilitation techniques on the life-table outcome curves [46].

Neural Net for Data Analysis

In recent years, neural net has become used more and more in medical science [48,49]. Neural net is a model that simplifies synaptic transmission of the neuron in a manner that can be handled by a computer. In rehabilitation medicine it has been used as a control algorithm [50,51], but neural net itself is potentially useful as a predictive algorithm as well. Because it can handle not only interval variables but also ordinal and even categorical variables, and because multicollinearity, which poses significant problems in the multiple regression method, is not a serious problem, it can be useful in prognostication studies in rehabilitation medicine. Sonoda et al. [52] used neural net in a preliminary prognostication study in stroke patients and found that it gave a better coefficient of determination as compared to traditional multiple regression analysis. Neural net and newer computer algorithms are increasingly used in the selection and construction of models from data. The further development of computer science will definitely provide us with a powerful tool in future outcome studies.

Cross-Validation

In his critical review of 33 outcome studies, Jongbloed [8] found that only 4 of the groups performed cross-validation of their findings. Cross-validation of the prediction rules derived from one study is indispensable to make the rules generalizable because the study sample of that particular study is not necessarily representative of all stroke patients. Often, internal validation through split-sample analysis is re-

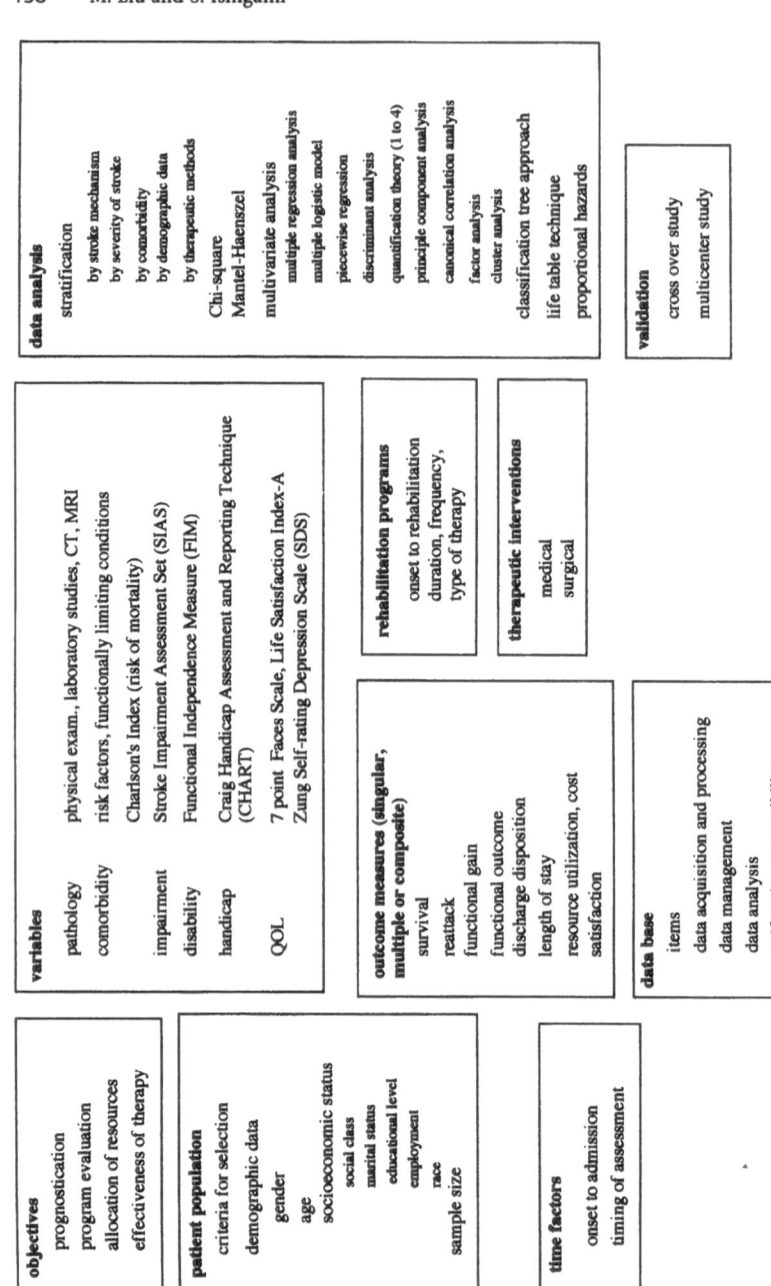

Fig. 2. The scope of stroke outcome research includes objectives of research, patient selection, time factors, measures (explanatory and outcome), database, therapy, and data analysis. Future outcome studies should follow well-designed and standardized protocols. CT, Computed tomography; MRI, magnetic resonance imaging; QOL, quality of life

ported, but unless the sample is derived from multicenter trials, it cannot be taken automatically as evidence of cross-validation. To minimize bias, the studies are preferably performed on a multicenter basis, and cross-validity is better confirmed in different population samples.

International Research

International research provides us with unique opportunities to compare different health care systems, clarify the problems in each country, and formulate strategies for improvement. In the area of stroke outcome research, several important international studies have been reported so far [53-55]. There are, however, some difficulties associated with international cooperative studies as pointed out by Anderson et al. [56].

First, differences in demographic characteristics are so significant that attempts to attribute variations in health care costs or outcomes to differences in health care financing and delivery systems are potentially misleading. Second, because culture can influence the choice of treatment options, international comparisons of illness patterns and response to illness can be misleading. Third, there are problems of instrument selection: measures with proven validity and reliability in one country are not necessarily valid and reliable in other cultures. There are also conceptual differences and problems of translation. To ensure that the same concept and nuance are translated to other languages, back-translation to the original language is recommended [56]. To further promote international research, it is necessary to explore and establish a sound methodology addressing its unique, inherent problems.

Conclusion

The scope of stroke outcome research can be schematized as in Fig. 2. There is an urgent need to develop a valid and reliable set of standardized measures of stroke pathology, comorbidity, impairment, disability, handicap, and life satisfaction that could be internationally used. Future outcome studies should follow well-designed and standardized protocols including patient selection, measures used, data acquisition, management, and analysis so that we can compare different studies on a common framework and generalize the conclusions. Furthermore, we need to promote international cooperative research that would provide us with a unique opportunity to compare different health care systems and achieve more insight into the problems related to stroke rehabilitation.

Acknowledgment. The authors sincerely thank Dr. Naoichi Chino, Professor, Department of Rehabilitation Medicine, Keio University School of Medicine, and Dr. John L. Melvin, Professor, Department of Physical Medicine and Rehabilitation, Temple University for their important suggestions and reviews of this manuscript.

References

1. World Health Organization (1980) International classification of impairments, disabilities, and handicap. Geneva

2. Hamilton BB, Granger CV, Sherwin FS, et al (1987) A uniform national data system for medical rehabilitation. In: Fuhrer MJ (ed) Rehabilitation outcomes: analysis and measurement. Brookers, Baltimore, pp 115–150
3. Granger CV, Hamilton BB (1992) The uniform data system for medical rehabilitation report of first admissions for 1992. Am J Phys Med Rehabil 73:51–55
4. Granger CV, Hamilton BB (1993) The uniform data system for medical rehabilitation report of first admissions for 1991. Am J Phys Med Rehabil 72:33–38
5. American Spinal Injury Association standards for neurological and functional classification of spinal cord injury (1992) American Spinal Injury Association, Chicago
6. American Heart Association (1991) Heart and stroke facts. American Heart Association, Washington, DC
7. Japanese Association of Rehabilitation Medicine (1994) The white paper of rehabilitation—toward the 21st century, 2nd edn. Ishiyaku, Tokyo, pp 240–243
8. Jongbloed L (1986) Prediction of function after stroke: a critical review. Stroke 17:765–776
9. Dombovy ML, Aandok BA, Basford JR (196) Rehabilitation for stroke: a review. Stroke 17:363–369
10. Task Force on Stroke Impairment, Stroke Disability, and Stroke Handicap (1990) Symposium recommendations for methodology in stroke outcome research. Stroke 21(suppl 2):68–73
11. Maklan CW, Greene R, Cummings MA (1993) Methodological challenges and innovations in patient outcomes research. Med Care 32(suppl):13–21
12. Fowler FJ, Cleary PD, Magaziner J, Patrick DL, Benjamin KL (1994) Methodological issues in measuring patient-reported outcomes: the agenda of the work group on outcomes assessment. Med Care 32(suppl):65–76
13. Nunnally JC, Bernstein IH (1994) Psychometric theory, 3rd edn. McGraw-Hill, New York, pp 1–30
14. Johnston MV, Keith RA (1993) Measurement standards for medical rehabilitation and clinical applications. Phys Med Clin North Am 4:417–449
15. Silverstein B, Fisher WP, Kilgore KM, Harley JP, Harvey RF (1992) Applying psychometric criteria to functional assessment in medical rehabilitation: II. Defining interval measures. Arch Phys Med Rehabil 73:507–518
16. Wilkin D, Hallam L, Doggett M-A (1992) Measures of need and outcome for primary health care. Oxford University Press, New York
17. Wright BD, Masters GN (1982) Rating scale analysis. MESA Press, Chicago
18. Kilgore KM, Fisher WP, Silverstein B, Harley JP, Harvey RF (1993) Application of Rasch analysis to the patient evaluation and conference system. Phys Med Clin North Am 4:493–515
19. Wade DT (1992) Measurement in neurological rehabilitation. Oxford University Press, New York
20. Kinkel WR (1990) Classification of stroke by neuroimaging technique. Stroke 21(suppl 2):7–8
21. Kinkel WR (1983) Computerized tomography in clinical neurology. In: Baker AB (ed) Clinical neurology. Philadelphia, Harper and Row, pp 1–115
22. Kinkel PR (1987) Nuclear magnetic resonance imaging in clinical neurology. In: Baker AB (ed) Clinical neurology. Philadelphia, Harper and Row, pp 1–68
23. Charlson ME, Pompei P, Ales KL, MacKenzie CR (1987) A new method of classifying prognostic comorbidity in longitudinal studies: development and validation. J Chronic Dis 40:373–383
24. Chino N, Sonoda S, Domen K, Saitoh E, Kimura A (1996) Stroke impairment assessment set (SIAS). In: Chino M, Melvin JL (eds) Functional evaluation of stroke patients. Springer, Tokyo, pp 19–31
25. Demeurisse G, Demol O, Robaye E (1980) Motor evaluation in vascular hemiplegia. Eur Neurol 19:382–389
26. Bohannon RW, Smith MB (1987) Interrater reliability of a modified Ashworth scale of muscle spasticity. Phys Ther 67:206–207

27. Tsuji T, Sonoda S, Domen K, Chino N (1994) The ADL structure of stroke patients in Japan; using functional independence measure. In: 7th World Congress of the International Rehabilitation Medicine Association, Washington, DC
28. Whiteneck GG, Charlifue SW, Gerhart KA, Overholser JD, Richardson GN (1992) Quantifying handicap: a new measure of long-term rehabilitation outcomes. Arch Phys Med Rehabil 73:519–526
29. Ware JE, Sherbourne CD (1992) The MOS 36 Item Short Form Health Survey. 1. Conceptual framework and item selection. Med Care 30:473–481
30. Neugarten BL, Havighurst RJ, Tobin SS (1961) The measurement of life satisfaction. J Gerontol 16:134–143
31. Cronbach LJ, Furby L (1970) How we should measure "change"—or should we? Psychol Bull 74:68–80
32. Falconer KA, Naughton BJ, Dunlop DD, Roth EJ, Strasser DC, Sinacore JM (1994) Predicting stroke inpatient rehabilitation outcome using a classification tree approach. Arch Phys Med Rehabil 75:619–625
33. Stineman MG, Escarce JJ, Goin JE, Hamilton BB, Granger CV, Williams SV (1994) A case-mix classification system for medical rehabilitation. Med Care 32:366–379
34. Data Management Service of the Uniform Data System for Medical Rehabilitation and the Center for Functional Assessment Research (1994) Guide for use of the uniform data set for medical rehabilitation, version 4. State University of New York, Buffalo
35. Wyatt JC, Altman DG, Heathfield HA, Pantin CFA (1994) Development of Design-Trial, a knowledge-based critiquing system for authors of clinical trial protocols. Comput Methods Programs Biomed 43:283–291
36. Armitage P, Berry G (1994) Statistical methods in medical research. 3rd edn. Blackwell, London, pp 178–181
37. Hayashi C (1950) On the quantification of phenomena from qualitative data from mathematico-statistical point of view. Ann Inst Stat Mat:3:69–98
38. Haga T (1984) Conversational data analysis system (in Japanese). Appl Stat 13:125–137
39. Domen K, Chino N, Sonoda S, Saitoh E, Kimura A (1991) Stroke impairment assessment set (SIAS)—a preliminary report. Arch Phys Med Rehabil 72:770
40. Kleinbaum DG (1994) Logistic regression. A self-learning text. In: Dietz K, Gail M, Krickeberg K, Singer B (eds) Statistics in the health sciences. Springer-Verlag, New York
41. Breiman L, Friedman JH, Olshen RA, Stone CJ (1984) Classification and regression trees. Wadsworth International Group, Belmont, CA
42. CART (1984) California Statistical Software, Lafayette, CA
43. Efron B, Tibshirani R (1991) Statistical data analysis in the computer age. Science 253:390–395
44. Lubinsky D (1994) Algorithmic speedups in growing classification trees by using an additive split criterion. In: Cheeseman P, Oldford RW (eds) Selecting models from data. Artificial intelligence and statistics 4. Lecture notes in statistics, vol 89. Springer-Verlag, New York, pp 435–444
45. Lutsko JF, Kuijpers B (1994) Simulated annealing in the construction of near-optimal decision trees. In: Cheeseman P, Oldford RW (eds) Selecting models from data. Artificial intelligence and statistics 4. Lecture notes in statistics, vol 89. Springer-Verlag, New York, pp 453–462
46. Reding MJ (1990) A model stroke classification scheme and its use in outcome research. Stroke 21(suppl 2):35–37
47. Armitage P, Berry G (1994) Statistical methods in medical research. 3rd edn. Blackwell, London, pp 470–472
48. Patil S, Henry JW, Rubenfire M, Stein PD (1993) Neural network in the clinical diagnosis of acute pulmonary embolism. Chest 104:1685–1689
49. Tu VJ, Guerriere MRJ (1993) Use of a neural network as a predictive instrument for length of stay in the intensive care unit following cardiac surgery. Comput Biomed Res 26:220–229
50. Holzreiter SH, Kohle ME (1993) Assessment of gait patterns using neural networks. J Biomech 26:645–651

51. Rosenbaum DA, Engelbrecht SE, Bushe MM, Loukopoulos LD (1993) A model for reaching control. Acta Psychol (Amst) 82:237–250

52. Sonoda S, Saitoh E, Tujiuchi K, Suzuki M, Domen K, Naoich C (1994) Application of neural net for outcome prediction in stroke patients. Presented at the 77th Kanto Rehabilitation Medicine Conference, Yokohama

53. Chino N, Anderson TP, Granger CV (1988) Stroke rehabilitation outcome studies: comparison of Japanese facility with 17 U.S. facilities. Int Disabil Stud 10:150–154

54. Chino N (1990) Efficacy of Barthel index in evaluating activities of daily living in Japan, the United States and United Kingdom. Stroke 21:64–65

55. Granger C, Aude M, Chino N, Fleury J, Frommelt P, Grimby G, Hagedoorn A, Hunter J, Lains J, Leszczynski J, Marossezky J, Minaire P, Tesio L (1994) Toward worldwide uniformity in functional assessment. In: 7th World Congress of the International Rehabilitation Medicine Association, Washington, DC

56. Anderson GF, Alonso J, Kohn LT, Black C (1994) Analyzing health outcomes through international comparison. Med Care 32:526–534

Index